Integrating Public Policy
into the Curriculum

Sally B. Solomon and Susan C. Roe, Editors

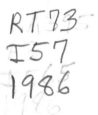
Pub. No. 15-1995

National League for Nursing • New York

PREFACE

The purpose of *Integrating Public Policy into the Curriculum* is to provide nursing faculty with the theoretical background and practical resources they need to teach public policy at the baccalaureate and graduate levels. The book provides a rationale for the inclusion of public policy in the curriculum, essays by prominent nursing educators on teaching strategies, a model course, a survey of current public policy courses, extensive lists of resources, and case studies for classroom use. An accompanying *Student Workbook* includes definitions of key concepts and terms in public policy as well as learning exercises to be used either independently or with the model course. Finally, a slide program, *Key Concepts in Public Policy,* provides basic information on government and health care policy in an easily grasped visual format. These three pieces of the program, used together or separately, will enable nursing faculty to implement a graduate-level public policy course or undergraduate curricular strand.

Numerous recent publications on policy and politics attest to the nursing profession's recognition of the importance of including these topics in the curriculum. Nurses have come to recognize that a knowledge of policy will enable them to explain their profession's needs and views to those who make decisions in local, state, and federal governments — decisions that affect nursing practice and the health of patients at the most basic level.

Although nurses are aware of the importance of policy in education and practice, there is still a shortage of faculty members prepared by experience and education to teach it. By providing both theoretical and practical information on policy, this book will be a first step in remedying this problem and thus will benefit students as well. The model course included in Chapter 3 will serve as a starting point.

Students' needs, and faculty members' expectations of them, of course differ at the baccalaureate, master's, and doctoral levels. Baccalaureate students need to acquire basic knowledge of policy and politics, familiarity with key terms and important government agencies, and awareness of leadership roles and career options open to nurses. Their needs are best served by inclusion of policy strands in other required courses, such as those on the health care system, leadership, and roles. Faculty members can select content from the model course as needed; the Basic Exercises in the *Student Workbook* are also designed for baccalaureate students. Successful completion of these exercises will demonstrate mastering of basic content in policy and politics for both baccalaureate and graduate students.

Master's level students have different needs. It is a premise of this book (and certainly an assumption of the editors) that all master's level nurses have been prepared to be leaders of the profession and that every master's program in nursing should offer a required course in health policy. Such courses will differ in emphasis, content, and structure according to the beliefs and abilities of the faculty, but students must master certain basic content. Because we believe both in the importance of teaching basic material and in allowing maximum flexibility to individual schools, the model course we present in Chapter 3 is designed as a series of independent modules, each covering an important content area. See Chapter 3 for suggestions about how to use the modules and about teaching methods.

This book begins with a stirring essay by Pamela Maraldo on the vital importance of preparing nurses to take an active role in health care policy and politics: "Nursing students must be taught that they have the power, the right, and the responsibility to influence health policy to change a system that is no longer working effectively." Chapter 2, by Donna Diers, shows how policy and politics affect the everyday lives of nurses and their patients and points out some of the many instances in which nurses have intervened successfully in policy making. Diers's essay broadens the definition of policy beyond the legislative process to include every aspect of nursing practice, with important implications for teaching.

Chapter 3 presents a model graduate public policy course based on the courses offered by a sample of graduate programs throughout the country. The course includes a detailed syllabus, learning objectives, and evaluation methods and is divided into seven modules that may be used individually or in combination. Chapter 4, by Barbara Dunn, Linda Hodges, and Judith Collins, reports the results of a curriculum survey of NLN-accredited master's programs. The authors found, among other things, a general acknowledgment among nursing educators of the importance of public policy and a shortage of faculty members prepared to teach it.

Chapter 5, by Sister Rosemary Donley, explores the politics of teaching public policy—the difficulties of making room for additional content in the curriculum and the skills needed to lobby successfully for inclusion of policy in the curriculum. Donley also discusses teaching strategies and ways of preparing faculty members to teach policy content. In Chapter 6, Jeffrey Merrill, Marcia Sass, and Stephen Somers pose challenging questions about the connection between research and public policy and perhaps challenge the assumptions of many in the academic world about the ways research influences policy.

Chapter 7, "Resources for Teaching Public Policy," by Diane McGivern, presents exhaustive discussion and listings of resources available to faculty members, including books, newspapers and news-letters, journals, government publications, organizations, audiovisual materials, and fellowships for students. Complete listings, including addresses and telephone numbers, are provided for all resources.

Chapter 8, by Susan Roe, sets out a theoretical framework for use of the case study method and explains the importance of this method for teaching public policy. The chapter includes two sample case studies (keyed to the model course in Chapter 3), suggestions for their use by students, and a reference list. Use of these timely case studies will force students to confront the dilemmas facing the nursing profession in a realistic way and make them aware of the complexity of the issues that face them in their practice every day.

This book is meant to be used with the accompanying workbook, *Key Concepts in Public Policy,* which is geared to the needs of bac-calaureate and graduate students and nurses in practice settings. The workbook includes both pen-and-pencil and experiential exercises designed to ensure that students acquire factual information as well as experience with the active role in policy. The Basic Exercises, intended for baccalaureate students, should be mastered by graduate students before they attempt the Advanced Exercises intended for them. Sug-gested answers to all exercises are provided, as well as resources for obtaining further information.

Other features of the *Student Workbook* include a discussion of key concepts in understanding policy and a comprehensive glossary of im-portant terms and policy-making bodies. The case studies included in this book are reproduced for the student's use, as is the resource list. Finally, the workbook includes additional small-group exercises that may be done in class.

The final component of these public policy learning materials, a color slide package with accompanying script, includes charts and diagrams that illustrate basic political concepts and key policy points. The slides can be used in educational settings by groups of students or faculty members, or in practice settings for inservice education. We have prepared these slides in the hope that they will fulfill what we see as a real need for audiovisual materials to illustrate basic content in the area of policy and politics.

We wish to thank the following people for providing us with information: Michael Hash, Health Policy Alternatives, Inc.; Karen Ehrnman, American College of Nurse-Midwives; and Susan M. Jenkins, legal counsel to the District of Columbia Nurses' Association. They were of great help to us in making sure our factual details were correct; however, we are of course responsible for the accuracy of the final publication. We also thank Elaine Silverstein, our editor at NLN, for her patience, perseverance, and guidance throughout this project, and the deans and faculties of nursing educational programs for participating in the survey that formed the basis for the model course.

Sally B. Solomon
Susan C. Roe

Contents

ABOUT THE AUTHORS

Judith B. Collins, MS, RN, is co-director, Health Policy Office, and associate professor, Schools of Nursing and Medicine, Virginia Commonwealth University/Medical College of Virginia, Richmond.

Donna Diers, MSN, FAAN, is professor, School of Nursing, Yale University, New Haven, Connecticut.

Sister Rosemary Donley, PhD, FAAN, is dean of nursing, The Catholic University of America, Washington, D.C.

Barbara H. Dunn, PhD, RN, is co-director, Health Policy Office, and adjunct associate professor, School of Nursing, Virginia Commonwealth University/Medical College of Virginia, Richmond; and visiting associate professor, School of Nursing, University of Virginia, Charlottesville.

Linda C. Hodges, EdD, RN, is acting director of the graduate program and associate professor, College of Nursing, Medical University of South Carolina, Charleston.

Pamela Maraldo, PhD, RN, is executive director, National League for Nursing, New York.

Diane O. McGivern, PhD, RN, is associate professor, School of Nursing, University of Pennsylvania, Philadelphia.

Jeffrey C. Merrill, MPH, is vice-president, The Robert Wood Johnson Foundation, Princeton, New Jersey.

Susan C. Roe, MS, RN, is a consultant specializing in health care policy, education, and personnel development, Phoenix, Arizona.

Marcia M. Sass, ScD, RN, is executive director, Study of Long-Term Outcome of Very Low Birthweight Infants, University of Pennsylvania, Philadelphia.

Sally B. Solomon, MSN, RN, is director, Division of Public Policy and Research, National League for Nursing, New York.

Stephen A. Somers, PhD, is a program officer, The Robert Wood Johnson Foundation, Princeton, New Jersey.

1

THE IMPORTANCE OF POLICY IN THE NURSING CURRICULUM

Pamela J. Maraldo

There is no topic of more vital importance to our students than health policy. At this point in our growth and development as a profession, a thorough knowledge of health policy is just as essential to our students as an understanding of the side effects of penicillin. In fact, it may be more essential. Some in nursing will immediately take umbrage at this statement. They would assert that research or clinical proficiency or the quality of nursing care should undoubtedly precede health policy in the order of important topics taught to nursing students today.

Yet it is easy to recall numerous events of the past two decades or so that have repeatedly demonstrated the superior importance of health policy in the hierarchy of things nursing students need to know.

In his recent work *The Social Transformation of American Medicine*, Paul Starr recounts the tilt toward hospitals and medical schools that has persisted in health policy for no substantive reason. He asserts that health policy debates over HMOs, PSROs, health planning, and national health insurance have ebbed and flowed for the past 15 years at the behest of the American Medical Association. Starr's description of the origins of the Medicare program make the point:

In setting up Medicare, Congress and the Administration were acutely concerned to gain the cooperation of the doctors and hospital. As a result, the administration of Medicare was lodged in the private insurance systems (Blue Cross, Blue Shield) originally established to suit provider interests. The federal government surrendered direct control of the program and its costs to appease organized medicine. Medicare and its retrospective system of reimbursement, and physician dominion over the program, have been charged by many as the major culprits for the uncontrollable health care costs for the past 20 years.

Once again, politics, not research, wisdom, or facts, was the chief health policy maker of the Medicare program.

For nurses the list of politically driven decisions in health policy is endless. During the Carter administration, when a heightened awareness of escalating health care costs was a high priority, the administration took the position that there was an adequate supply of nurses in the country, in the face of a dire nursing shortage. The administration held firmly to this stance despite the many, many research studies that presented facts to the contrary. The administration was attempting to reduce federal spending, and among the many special interests clamoring for funds, nurses were considered to be a force with little resistance. Politics, not research, was the driving force behind the administration's immovable stance.

Studies abound as to the cost savings that would accrue to the health care system if nurses replaced physicians in certain primary-care capacities. (The quality of care delivered by the nurses has been shown to be as good as or better than that of physicians.) Yet national health policy reports caution against the future use of nurse practitioners because of the anticipated oversupply of physicians.

The extraordinary amount of money spent on biomedical research annually is another glaring example of the highly political nature of health policy decision making. Despite the fact that many of the 15 leading causes of death in the United States have little or no sensitivity to medical treatment, such as alcoholism, homicide, and suicide, as a nation we spend $10 billion annually on biomedical research and consider research into life-style and the social sciences "soft" and unscientific.

In light of continuous and persistent examples of the highly political nature of decision making in health care, if we nurses expect to hold firm to the commitment that we exist to meet the health needs of the public, a thorough command of health policy must be our overriding concern. We can succeed in educating the most talented nurses in our institutions of higher learning so that they emerge with effective analytic skills, good basic mathematic ability, a fine grasp of research design, and excellent writing skills. But if they have no command of health policy and how it is developed, these talented professionals are destined to suffer from the reality shock and impotence that has frustrated and disillusioned us all for many years. Without better grounding in health policy, we will continue to send our graduates into a health care system that not only fails to appreciate their ability to analyze and think but does not allow them to do so.

The study of health policy must be broadly defined to include its most important instruments—power, politics, and economic interests. These tools of health policy making are used to carve out the decisions we in health care live by. As the cloud of economic uncertainty continues to darken our health care system, political battles will increase in number and intensity. Because the largest purchaser of health care is the federal government (through the Medicare program), and because government spending on health care will continue to be limited in the foreseeable future, power struggles over scarcer and scarcer resources will inevitably escalate. In a climate of this nature, the nursing profession is in danger of losing ground, because the levers of power in health care are not under our control.

We teach our nursing students that nursing is an autonomous profession. Indeed, its theoretical underpinnings and conceptual frameworks constitute an autonomous body of knowledge. But a venture into the real world of health care delivery quickly demonstrates that nursing is, in most cases, not autonomous at all. And so, far from ensuring that the health care needs of people are met, we nurses have little to say about them.

Of course, there has been progress. During the past decade we have seen nurses rise to high-ranking positions in health care, as well as in government and industry. We have seen a nurse administer the awesome Medicare budget as head of the Health Care Financing Administration, we have seen a nurse become deputy chief of staff to the majority leader of the Senate, and we have seen a nurse become the chief operating officer of one of the largest, most prestigious medical centers in the country. Other successes for nurses include the passage of a bill to establish a National Institute of Nursing through both houses of Congress (even though in the final analysis it received a presidential veto) and the enactment of several laws providing third-party reimbursement to nurses.

Yet there is a long way to go. In all but exceptional cases, we nurses do not have enough control over the nursing care we deliver to patients to ensure its effectiveness or its quality. Despite our large numbers, we have an all but insignificant involvement in the policies that govern our health care institutions. In broad national health policy discussions, nursing's voice is conspicuously absent. For example, we in health care have a new system of hospital financing that is revolutionizing our health care system. Were nurses, represented by any collective group, involved in any of the debates or discussions that resulted in the DRG system of hospital financing? No, we were not. Home health care is very popular these days as the humanistic, cost-effective alternative to acute-care hospitalization. Are we nurses considered the predominant providers in home care any longer? No, we are not. Social workers consider social workers to be predominant; respiratory therapists consider respiratory therapy to be predominant; physical therapists consider physical therapy to be predominant; and physicians see the growing popularity of this form of care and are moving quickly into this arena. Prevention is widely touted as the great hope for saving untold dollars by forestalling costly hospitalizations and improving the quality of American life through exercise, better nutrition, and stress reduction. Curricula in schools of nursing are built around the theme of prevention. Yet are we nurses involved in the numerous prevention initiatives in health policy and industry throughout the country? No, we are not.

We nurses have always delivered care independently to patients in their homes, in their workplaces, in the community. Then, with the growth and proliferation of the medical industrial complex, nursing was swallowed up and split into a plethora of therapies and specialties and nursing's domain was withered away.

We need a nursing liberation movement. We in nursing need social reform in our profession to change the way we see ourselves. Such a movement, like the women's liberation movement, would socialize us to realize our true worth to society and the power we have as a body politic. Most importantly, a liberation movement would inspire us to wield the power we have to improve health care in the nation. At present, we nurses do little to oppose medical policies that we do not approve of. We strongly believe, as a group, that there are limits to medical science; that there are clearly preferable alternatives to drugs and surgery for promoting health and well-being. As a society we see ubiquitous evidence that a sickness-oriented medical system is far too costly and too palliative in its promises to cure the sick, yet we seem immobilized and unable to alter it. There are formidable political barriers to mount in setting out to change the health care system. But the greatest problem we nurses have lies in our inability to engender and maintain the belief among ourselves that we have the power to change things. Efforts to remedy this lack of political strength and conviction must be rooted in our students. Nursing students of today must be taught that they have the power, the right, and the responsibility to influence health policy to change a system that is no longer working effectively.

Nurses have many potential solutions to the problems that plague our health care system: the ability to offer lower cost alternatives, the ability to provide the humanistic sensitivity that patients crave, and the ability to provide great continuity to patients as they move through a morass of fragmented services where they meet frustration and isolation.

It is obvious that in order to exert enough influence on health policy to change a woefully inadequate system, we must learn to mobilize our political strength. An undertaking of this magnitude has to begin by cultivating in our students what John Kenneth Galbraith refers to as "bimodal symmetry" in the nursing profession. This means that in order to effect external change, a group must first have internal cohesion. To the extent that a body politic can minimize internal dissension, it will succeed in having greater external influence in policy-making spheres. This, as Galbraith describes it, is the invariable feature of all exercise of organized power: that individuals adjust their own aims and goals to the common purposes of the group, and from this internal exercise of power comes the ability of the group to impose its will externally. If internal cohesion is high, the chance of influencing external public policy is high. Of course, the antithesis of this situation is an oft-stated political axiom. As Galbraith puts it, nothing so weakens the external power of a group or organization as the undisciplined expression of dissenting views from within. This is the bimodal symmetry of internal and external power.

The achievement of this bimodal symmetry must be our mission. Students of nursing must be taught to understand the profession's overarching need for cohesion. No one is likely to question the need for the basics of health policy in the curriculum: how a bill becomes a law, the separation of powers, and how health care agencies are reimbursed. These are important subjects, but they do not get to the heart of the health policy matter. Our teachers and our leaders in nursing must explain and ingrain in our students a knowledge of the use of power. Practical political discussions must be held in nursing's health policy classes. Students should discuss live health policy issues and practice the generation of new strategies, with a mind toward really winning once they leave the classroom. Students should be taught the paramount importance of unity and cohesion, and in the classroom these instruments of influence should be deeply fostered. Our nursing students must be strongly motivated to act in unison to work toward better health care delivery upon leaving our institutions of higher learning. They must be motivated to go out and do it: to make a difference in the way health care is delivered. If we can instill this ability and drive in tomorrow's nursing students, we will have successfully taught them not only how to make health policy but also how to be good nurses.

2

POLICY AND POLITICS: IMPLICATIONS FOR CURRICULUM

Donna Diers

Policy has become one of nursing's hot topics. Witness the number of new publications that highlight the word, the number of times *policy* appears in convention programs, and the increasing attention it commands in curricular planning. This heightened interest proves our growing sophistication. As more nurses take leading positions both within the health care field and outside of it—positions that bring us into contact with policy and policy makers—we realize that we must boost our participation in policy forums. And we are starting to notice that, as the largest single group within the health care system, nursing has been less than well represented in policy making at the federal, state, local, and institutional levels.

UNDERSTANDING WHY

The point of learning about or teaching policy is to equip nurses to feel less victimized by what they see as a random world. The world may not always be rational, but it is not random. Things happen as they do for reasons. Understanding how and why things happen is the first step in forming or changing policy. The study of policy, then, is the study of decision making. Perhaps put that way, it loses some of its mystery and seems more obviously linked to the other kinds of decision making we teach and learn through the nursing curriculum. When nurses learn to trust and to mine our clinical information, we can make a special contribution to policy.

Teaching or learning policy means learning the process of discovery. Many nursing content areas cannot be taught through discovery—they must be set down as procedure. For example, an instructor cannot allow students to contaminate operating rooms by not wearing masks while they learn aseptic technique. So we make rules and insist that students memorize them. But in teaching policy, the process of discovery works. Consider this example:

A hospital chief executive officer has just announced that, next year, no new nursing positions will be created and unfilled positions will be frozen. A staff nurse, who is already working double shifts, feels victimized by an insensitive and inattentive administration. Her complaints to the supervisor do not seem to accomplish anything, nor do the supervisor's complaints to administrators, which convinces the nurse that the situation is caused by random, arbitrary decisions in which nurses had no voice.

Suppose the nurse begins to wonder why. Suppose she asks about the financial aspects of the problem. She would learn that the hospital has a problem with its regulatory agency and current yearly budget because the census is under what was budgeted. Why, she asks. Because fewer patients are being admitted, and those who are admitted are not staying as long as they used to (and this is before prospective payment). Why? Because a new hospital in town is courting surgeons with early operating times to build its clientele. And the new chief of surgery in her hospital has decreed that the first priority on operating room time will go to the full-time faculty of the school of medicine. Annoyed, the community doctors are taking their patients to the new hospital.

Pressing further, she might discover that workers in several local industries are on strike and that unemployment is up, so many people are not seeking needed hospital care because they cannot afford it. Finally, pressing to the limit, the nurse might learn that some physicians find the nursing care in her hospital to be below par, primarily due to understaffing, and therefore do not want their patients admitted there, which only exacerbates the problem (Diers, 1979).

Students who choose to study this issue might stop with the realization that planned staffing cuts are a policy problem, with the policy value being to control the hospital's deficit. A staff nurse, on the other hand, might take the policy issue further to organize ideas and talent to help the hospital increase its census.

Policy and Clinical Decisions

At an institutional level, policy is evident not only in such management issues but also in clinical decisions. Analyses of clinical policy issues fit easily into nursing curricula. For example, hospital procedure manuals have guidelines for how to handle a case of suspected transfusion reaction. Among the things nurses are instructed to do is to get a urine sample, which can be a problem with a patient who is worried and shivering and who is sick enough to be getting blood in the first place. Tracking down this policy, the nurse would discover that it was written into the manual 30 years ago, when there were no quick and easy ways to determine whether the patient was hemolyzing, which is the reason for the urine sample.

These kinds of policy concerns surround us. It would be a service to students, as well as to the facility, to track a few of them down to see whether the original value still applies. For example, an educator could suggest that students find out why nursing shifts run from 7:00 A.M. to 3:00 P.M., from 3:00 P.M. to 11:00 P.M., and from 11:00 P.M. to 7:00 A.M. The policy issue that first determined this has been lost in the mists of hospital organization and labor laws, but, at one time, there was a real reason for this timing. When nursing shifts were reduced from twelve hours—7:00 A.M. to 7:00 P.M.—to eight hours, 7:00 A.M. was simply kept as the beginning point. Why? Probably because that's more or less when the sun comes up.

Searching for Data

Discovering the reasons for policy involves discovering the data on which policies are based. However, sometimes there are no data —just someone's idea of what should be. That occurs at the level of public policy as politics; at the level of clinical work, many practices have become policy for less than rational reasons.

For example, in this country the semisitting position is the common position for labor and delivery. No data demonstrate that this position is better for the woman or for the baby; in fact, recent data suggest that It causes more lacerations and longer second-stage labor and that it allows the woman less feeling of control over her body (Vedam &

Golay, 1985). Why, then, do we continue to use it? We do it because it is convenient for the birth attendant, a fact discovered by a French barber-surgeon in the 1700s. It makes doing pelvic exams, applying forceps, and generally taking charge of the woman's body easier. Hospitals have sometimes declared that only the semisitting position will be allowed, which is a strong example of policy not backed by data.

Of course, policy occasionally changes because of data. For instance, after surgery in the past, patients had to spend ten days in bed to allow the blood to thicken up again. It did indeed thicken, and thrombi occurred, so the policy was changed to encourage early ambulation.

Discovering policy begins simply with not taking things for granted. And if the first task in learning about policy is discovering the policy underpinnings for clinical exigencies, the second might be learning to distinguish among the types of arguments used in policy discussions or in political maneuvering.

DISCOVERING RATIONALE

In 1979, legislators in Oregon wrote a bill to permit certain properly qualified nurses to prescribe drugs. In reporting on the fate of the legislation, Dunn describes the resistance of the Oregon Medical Association (OMA), whose leaders said nurses did not have the educational qualifications to hold prescriptive authority. Dunn says, "at times OMA arguments were couched in condescending language and implied that nurses were somehow 'brainless little girls' " (Dunn, 1983). The Oregon nurses could have become inflamed by such arguments and pinned their battle on defending their intellects and their roles. They did not, partly because the proposed law required formal pharmacology preparation and continuing education, and, more importantly, because the issue was not how smart the nurses were, it was money and competition. So the Oregon Nurses' Association assembled data on such things as cost effectiveness, and the bill passed.

Money is behind so many policy and political issues that it is useful to look for its influence. For example, in the controversy about substituting practical nurses or aides for licensed professional nurses, it would not help for nurses to argue that RNs are better than LPNs or aides. Nor would it be a good use of our time to try to make tricky distinctions in conceptual or intellectual territory between RNs and others. The policy issue isn't RNs versus others, it's money. Many policy makers consider RNs more expensive; some have even alleged that the higher the proportion of RNs in a staff, the more trouble they make for the administration. Effective counterarguments use existing data to prove that RNs, being more versatile than any other group, can do their own work as well as that of others, which is cost-effective. More importantly, with the early discharge incentives created by prospective payment, a less well-prepared staff cannot accomplish the assessment, management, discharge planning, and patient teaching required for early discharge (Diers, 1985).

POLICY VERSUS POLITICS

Distinguishing among policy agendas is one kind of learning. Distinguishing between political strategies and policy agendas is another. Policy deals with shoulds and oughts; politics conditions, and sometimes impedes, both policy development and implementation. Politics is the use of power to persuade or otherwise change.[4] Policy is based in values, goals, or principles, even when those values may represent idiosyncratic bias. According to Milio, policy involves "identifying an issue as a proper sphere for . . . action and deciding what that action will be." Politics, then, is the "give and take" of negotiation (Milio, 1984). Politics is reactive; policy is proactive.

Most nursing literature about policy assumes that it can only be made in the context of government, particularly legislation, where votes count and the orthodox political process applies. But policy has wide application and even more narrow local application. Policy already exists in the curriculum, and efforts might be made simply to elevate it to consciousness rather than to try to squeeze new content in at the expense of clinical work, research, and theory.

The case of entry into practice helps pinpoint the distinction between policy and politics. The move to make the BSN the minimum qualification for professional licensure may have lost its policy goal to political interests. The debate now deals only with educational credentials. Had the position been conceived as a policy thrust, its "rightness" would be clear. A policy statement on this topic might say that nursing is complicated work and that the American people deserve experienced and intellectually able practitioners to deliver care and to humanize institutions. To produce such nurses, education should include not only carefully supervised clinical experience but also change theory, theories of health and disease, and all the rest. Then nurses would be properly equipped to meet the policy goal. One way to guarantee that the public's policy interests are met is to require evidence of such preparation for licensure. Note that I have not specified degree or other credentials.

Putting the policy issue this way makes clear the rather limited agenda that has occupied nursing since 1965 and has caused us to fight each other in public forums. Concern surrounding the "1985 proposal" has been converted into political concern—who has the loudest voice and the most votes (Diers, 1985). Barbara Stevens characterizes the initial failure of the state of New York to pass the BSN bill as "a failure to differentiate between political decision-making and intellectual ideas" (Stevens, 1985). Perhaps because the "ideas" were not cast as policy points, they remained remote from the political process. And if the policy goals had been called that, the resistance to the notion of grandfathering, which Stevens points out has been characteristic of every other profession's upward strivings, might not have been so severe. Finally, if the policy goal had been articulated, the legislature might not have been in the untenable position of having to decide between future professional advancement and the votes of the 80 percent of existing nurses who did not hold a BSN.

Another current example of the difference between politics and policy is the proposal for a National Institute of Nursing. Basically, what has happened is that the politics of the proposal determined the policy. The proposal for an institute, to be located within the National Institutes of Health, came from the office of a Republican congressman from Illinois. In 1984, when the proposal came up, the Republicans were thought to have a "gender gap," and, as Dumas and Felton guessed would happen, an up-and-coming congressman wanted to make his name by doing something for the 1 in 44 women voters who are nurses (Dumas & Felton, 1984). But since the political proposal, in the form of a bill, did not have the benefit of advance discussion in the nursing community, the policy issue was overtaken by the need for political activity. Policy issues were raised in the course of that activity—did nurses want to separate research from other functions in the federal funding system, would nursing research be better or less well served by its placement with other research in NIH, and so on. By then, nurses were in a position in which public infighting would not have been wise but in which public debate was no longer possible.

The NIH case teaches us how uncontrollable and how random politics can be, and that we should avoid flat-out political maneuvers we did not start. What is now apparent is that politicians do not have much interest in giving nursing a place in NIH—nursing is not that big a political coin, especially with its minute budget for research. What explains the political force is a young congressman's ambition and the need to trade support for various pet projects. Therefore, the institute issue will be settled outside of nursing's own politics, and perhaps outside of our interest, because nursing has become a token to be handed around in trade.

There are examples of the randomness of policy making as well. The reason we allegedly have a physician surplus is a case in point. Representative Paul Rogers, then chair of the House committee dealing with medical manpower, was called by a constituent who complained that he had recently had a long wait in a hospital emergency department. The constituent attributed the wait to a lack of doctors. Rogers told the story in hearings on manpower legislation and convinced his colleagues that they should do something about the physician shortage. One of Rogers's colleagues asked him how many doctors ought to be put in the hopper. The congressman turned to an aide, who grabbed a number out of the air—50,000—and that became the target.

Politics, including the basics—how law is made, the role of regulation, and so on—is neither difficult to understand nor to teach. In fact, there are several good books and many articles in the nursing literature from which to draw. The only mistake to avoid in reading this material is to think that policy is made only as "public" policy— the agendas of governments or government agencies. In fact, policy is made in many places and for many reasons, and nurses have the chance to participate more widely than we might at first believe.

Policy Makers

Policy is made in the courts, for instance, where legal judgments in one jurisdiction may have profound effects in others. Consider the case of the Missouri nurse practitioners, which ended with a state Supreme Court decision that the nurses involved were not practicing beyond the scope of their practice act by fitting diaphragms and examining patients. Before that case was settled, a similar case had been raised in another state. When the Missouri decision was rendered, the plaintiffs in the other case withdrew their charge.

Policy is also made in the private sector. For example, the decision of the Kellogg Foundation to support the National Council of State Boards of Nursing took the state boards out from under both of the two professional organizations with prior interest. That means the council no longer has a constituency to call on, and it is no accident that several states are now reconsidering the national state board examination as their credential for entry into practice.

Bureaucrats also make policy, sometimes randomly, and sometimes in ways that work for us. For instance, a Connecticut Department of Health official once decided that nurse-midwives could not sign birth certificates. He apparently reasoned that, since nurse-midwives were not then separately licensed, they did not exist. Nothing terrible happened if a nurse-midwife did sign the certificate as birth attendant, but the lack of credibility bothered the nurse-midwives. However, the official's decision turned out to work for us. When it came time for us to push for legal recognition of nurse-midwifery, those in opposition looked for facts to show how unsafe nurse-midwives were. They hunted through birth certificates to track infant mortality, birth weight, and complications, but no data were available. They could not even find out how many babies nurse-midwives had delivered, which put skids under the opposition.

Incorporating Clinical Wisdom

The most important kind of learning about policy, however, is learning how to make clinical wisdom accessible and meaningful to policy formulation. Policy should depend on data. Data for policy making are gathered from existing information, summarized with a particular question in mind. The existing data are produced by paper forms or by electronic counting systems, so the kind of paper form or data system in place may determine policy. It is to our advantage to pay attention to the development of such data-gathering systems.

For example, for years, in nearly every hospital and on every shift, nurses have classified patients into categories of acuity. That information was used for staffing subsequent shifts by attaching a staffing algorithm to patient condition. But then the paper forms were discarded and no permanent records of nurses' impressions of patients' conditions were kept.

When DRGs were put in place nurses panicked, because, in some cases, a DRG did not seem to define the consumption of nursing resources accurately. Now, as hospitals scramble to set up data retrieval systems by which to argue that the present DRG-fixed price per case does not reflect their case mix, nursing acuity and intensity have importance they did not have before.

There are several other kinds of policy issues here as well. For instance, Maine has passed legislation mandating that the cost of nursing service in institutions be shown on hospital bills. Some nurses have worried about the wisdom of the move, for we have historically had trouble justifying why we do what we do and why we have the right or the intelligence to do it. And now we are being asked not just to justify those things but also why it costs what it does. Nursing's policy point here might be what we have said for years: that nursing is an independent profession, a set of activities and theories and practices that has intellectual and clinical autonomy, and that our authority in institutions does not match our responsibility and accountability. This mismatch occurs in nursing economic invisibility; we cannot have it both ways. We can never claim the role we want—the role of authority to determine our own practice—until we can see what the work is. The only way to see that is to figure out how much of it there is and what it costs.

Therein lies the tricky policy point, and its solution will depend heavily on clinical wisdom. Should the economic definition of nursing be in terms of what nurses do—tasks or activities or minutes—or what nurses think? The answer is the latter, because it is closer to the reality. Counting tasks or minutes is not a good way to say what nursing is, much less how good it is.

Is it possible to devise a policy-relevant system of costing out nursing that taps how nurses think? Of course it is, and some already exist. For example, some nursing acuity measures rank patients from less to more ill and make the logical assumption that sicker patients need and get more care. Edward Halloran at University Hospitals of Cleveland has taken this system a step further and devised a checklist of nursing diagnoses, which, when taken together, could measure nursing resource consumption. However, Halloran's measure depends on the policy perspective that assumes that professional nurses pay attention to what patients need and deliver that service. RIMs (resource intensity measures), or other systems that define nursing by task or by minutes, will not be in our best interest in the long run because tasks or minutes can be cut from budgets; thinking cannot.

An internal policy issue could also benefit from clinical wisdom. The American Nurses' Association's Social Policy Statement, if not exactly "public policy," is certainly professional organization policy. It includes the language of the New York State Nurse Practice Act, which defines nursing as "diagnosing human responses to actual or potential health problems" (ANA, 1980). Some nurses, myself included, are concerned with that language, which originally had a policy point that may now have changed.

When the New York State Nurses' Association wrote that definition into its practice act in 1972, it was the novel to have the word *diagnosis* used in conjunction with nursing, and it was a great leap forward. The language is now often interpreted to mean that the only thing nurses do is diagnose human responses, which leaves out much of both traditional and new nursing functions. This policy issue surfaces: Should a definition of nursing be restrictive and confining, or enabling? And what is the purpose of definition? Practice acts are an extension of the state's police function, designed to protect the public. Yet they can also restrain the practice of individuals if they do not anticipate professional growth and development and if they do not make clinical sense. The New York State Nurse Practice Act, from which the social policy statement wording was taken, was intended to allow nurses to diagnose something, with language broad enough to be encompassing. To restrict the practice of nursing only to diagnosing human responses, among other things, eliminates the practice of psychiatric nursing as nursing, for there the "human response" is also the disease. It does not make clinical sense as policy.

Nurses will have endless opportunities to use clinical wisdom to influence public policy, especially while policy continues to focus on costs of care. Nurses are the only ones who know what really goes on in hospitals, nursing homes, and other total-care institutions. We are also the only ones who know the entire network of services outside of institutions into which people who have needs could be plugged. What we have to learn is how to articulate our clinical knowledge to policy makers.

When we come to value clinical work for its potential contribution to policy, the hesitancy we feel about participating in policy will disappear. When we learn how to speak "policy," in addition to "politics," the connection between the work we are trained and educated to do as nurses and policy matters becomes clear. As I've mentioned, policy deals with shoulds and oughts and therefore is close to ethics and moral decision making. Our intellectual and clinical tradition in nursing is to pay serious attention to those issues of value and to know how to protect them. Teaching policy, then, does not have to be different from teaching clinical decision making or research or anything else we teach now. Discovering the whys of the way the world operates, whether the issue is physiology or management, is central to teaching practice, and having policy as a curriculum thread might only mean taking what we presently do a step further and questioning the reasons behind things.

Policy is slow; it moves in tiny increments because it deals with large issues. People resist changes in values, which is what policy is, even more than changes in power, which is what politics is. The first step in policy making is simply "getting on the agenda" (Lindblom, 1980). When potential new policy runs counter to entrenched ideas or outdated values—as is often the case in nursing issues—getting on to policy agendas will be difficult. This calls for studying history, particularly contemporary history, that deals with themes and issues, rather than with people or dates.

TEACHING POLICY

Teaching policy, or putting it in the curriculum, then, is mostly a matter of deciding what to teach. I have discussed what is important about policy. The more policy can be understood as part of practice, the better it will be taught and the more understandable it will be to students.

At the undergraduate level, policy teaching might concentrate on policy as one of the contexts for clinical practice and on policy as management or system organization. At the graduate level, policy analysis, data strategies, and subtleties of group interactions might be highlighted. Teaching policy is teaching process, since all there is to be said about policy in health care is too vast to be absorbed by anyone. Therefore, teaching ought to lay the principles of analyzing policy and politics with the hope that students will use the principles when the need arises.

Policy is probably best taught from cases, because case method parallels policy process. Cases can be constructed on nearly any issue, for any level of student. Tracking down the rituals of practice as a policy issue, for example, provides a long list. Thinking about what nurses participate in will produce more: DNR orders, substitutability issues, collective bargaining, staffing ratios, participation in research on human subjects, malpractice, and the *respondeat superior* doctrine are just a few. Of course, the issues of third-party reimbursement, practice acts, funding for nursing programs, licensure, prescriptive authority, and the government's role in directing developments in practice, from the creation of new roles for nurses to restraint of trade, all provide cases to explore.

Prescribing particular courses, objectives, pedagogical strategies, or how much of what to teach is not the purpose of this chapter. However, I caution that, just because policy is hot right now and offers something new to the old nursing curricula, we should not get so infatuated with it that we lose sight of what it is—a context, nothing more, a context to be used when it helps move forward what we are here for—the delivery of human service.

REFERENCES

American Nurses' Association. (1980). *Nursing: A social policy statement.* Kansas City, MO: ANA.

Diers, D. (1979). Lessons on leadership. *Image, 11*(3), 67–71.

Diers, D. (1985). Policy and politics. In D. J.Mason & S. W. Talbott (Eds.), *Political action handbook for nurses.* Menlo Park, CA: Addison-Wesley.

Dumas, R., & Felton, G. (1984). Should there be a National Institute for Nursing? *Nursing Outlook, 32*(1), 16–22.

Dunn, A. M. (December 1983). Nurse activism in Oregon politics. *Nurse Practitioner, 80*, 54–56.

Fagin, C. (1982). The economic value of nursing research. *American Journal of Nursing, 82*, 1844–1849.

Lindblom, C. (1980). *The policy making process* (2d ed.). Englewood Cliffs, NJ: Prentice-Hall.

Milio, N. (1984). The realities of policy making—Can nurses have an impact? *Journal of Nursing Administration, 14*(3), 18–23.

Stevens, B. (1985). Nursing, politics, and policy formulation. In R. R. Wieczorek (Ed.), *Power, politics, and policy in nursing.* New York: Springer.

Vedam, S., & Golay, J. (1985). *Effectiveness of the squatting position in labor.* Unpublished master's thesis, Yale University School of Nursing, New Haven, Connecticut.

3

PUBLIC POLICY CURRICULA: PAST AND PRESENT PRACTICES AND FUTURE DIRECTIONS

Sally B. Solomon and Susan C. Roe

Because they occupy a key position at the point of delivery and have the most sustained contact with clients, nurses have a distinct advantage in shaping the health care environment. Clinical expertise is not enough to face the newly created challenges. To be effective leaders in health care policy, nurses must augment their clinical expertise with knowledge and skills in health care policy and politics.

This chapter focuses on how policy courses can be developed and integrated into nursing curricula. A historical and conceptual framework based on the linkage between curriculum development and the nurse's role provides a rationale for including health care policy in nursing curricula. The chapter provides a synopsis of current trends in nursing public policy curricula based on a convenience sample of undergraduate and graduate programs. Finally, an outline of a model health care policy course at the master's level is presented as a guide to integrating public policy into nursing curricula.

CONCEPTUAL FRAMEWORK

There exists in nursing education a well-established principle that the nursing curriculum influences the role that nurses play in the health care system. Similarly, current nursing practice guides faculty in the planning of curricula. This curriculum–role linkage explains the critical interaction between the integration of public policy into nursing curricula and nursing's needed leadership role in the health care policy arena. If nurses are to assume the role of change agent, preparation for this role must include deliberate placement of public policy into the curricula.

Examining the nursing process for its fullest potential includes an understanding of the economic, social, and political forces that influence client behavior. Reimbursement mechanisms, government-subsidized programs, and fiscal constraints are examples of critical issues that influence the way in which clients interact with the health care system. As a result, these issues need to be recognized by nursing as legitimate practice concerns and therefore integrated into nursing curricula and nursing care.

HISTORICAL FRAMEWORK

A glance at the history of nursing reveals that health care policy has a precedence and a historical place in nursing for both role development and curriculum content. Today's growing popularity of public policy for the nursing profession marks the return of an issue that had been a fundamental part of nursing practice and education.

In the nineteenth century, Florence Nightingale's advancement of nursing through hospital reform, and subsequent applications of her ideas to public health settings, required political savvy. These early examples of influencing policy signified the origins of nursing as a political force. However, one could argue that while Nightingale was a visionary in terms of health reform she was bound by the socioeconomic values of her era. These values limited the extent to which women who were nurses could rise to powerful positions within the male-dominated society. Consequently, Nightingale used strategies in attaining her goals that placed nursing in a structure that suited the times. However, this subordinate placement of nursing within the health care hierarchy has been an everpresent obstacle to the nursing profession (Ehrenreich & English, 1973).

In general, the development of nursing education and practice in the United States closely followed the Nightingale model. Consequently, American nurses in the late nineteenth and early twentieth centuries faced predicaments similar to those of their British colleagues in terms of their status as women in the health care hierarchy.

Many assume that nurses in the early twentieth century were closely aligned with the women's suffrage movement. As a group, nurses were not committed to the social feminism that was often associated with the suffragist activities. In many ways this parallels the relationship between nursing and the women's movement of the 1970s and 1980s. Specifically, although many individual nurses subscribed to feminist ideals, collectively nurses have been reluctant to identify with the values associated with the women's movement (Lagemann, 1983).

At the same time, in the early twentieth century, collegiate nursing education emerged. It was believed that nurses should be educated in the social and economic factors that influence the client's total needs. There was a focus on developing community health programs and extending nursing education beyond the walls of the hospital (Bridgman, 1966). These collegiate nursing educators were forward thinkers and used the educational system to their advantage in shaping the future role of the nurse. In order to succeed, one may assume that they had an appreciation for policy and politics in higher education, the work place, and the health care system.

As nurses responded to the social injustices of the early twentieth century, they pioneered the establishment of agencies such as Lillian Wald's Henry Street Settlement. This was the clinical setting for the first public health nursing course, which was offered by Columbia (Frank, 1953). Integration of this new curriculum by Columbia, based on a change in nursing's role, clearly illustrated the curriculum–role linkage discussed earlier. Furthermore, nurses' prompt response as social reformers in the practice setting, followed by the concomitant reaction in nursing education, demonstrates another of nursing's accomplishments as a significant social and political force.

From the early twentieth century to World War II, nursing established itself as a viable provider of health care. Placement within the health care system had been accomplished, and now the focus shifted to areas such as licensure and standards of practice.

The post–World War II era was noted for the proliferation of hospital beds as a result of the Hill-Burton Act (1946) and the development of new technology. The federal government demonstrated its concern for social welfare through legislation that not only provided funds for hospital construction but also offered certain populations access to needed health care services (e.g., Medicare and Medicaid). The increase in the use of new technology, the focus on acute care, and the demand for nursing services led nursing education to concentrate on the development of clinical expertise, once again illustrating the link between curriculum and role.

By the late 1970s, spiraling health care costs forced all participants in the health care system to direct their attention to constraining costs. This placed health care policy high on the federal government's agenda. By the 1980s it has become apparent that if nursing is to thrive, it must prepare itself to participate in this new health care policy environment. Nursing education must respond by expanding beyond its clinical focus and providing opportunities for students to acquire expertise in health care policy.

Nursing programs across the country have begun to integrate public policy into their curricula using different approaches. In order to determine the extent of integration of public policy into nursing curricula, we conducted an informal telephone survey in the summer of 1985. Dunn, Hodges, and Collins conducted a similar and more extensive survey in 1985 of NLN-accredited master's programs. Their findings are summarized in Chapter 4.

THE TELEPHONE SURVEY

Twenty-one accredited nursing programs were included in a convenience sample based on geographic representation and the likelihood that the schools would have public policy components in their curricula. The survey consisted of questions on the appropriate placement of public policy in nursing curricula; course offerings, either within the department of nursing or elsewhere in the university; short- and long-term plans; the faculty's attitude toward the integration of public policy; and faculty and other teaching resources. In total, 18 programs from all four NLN geographic regions were surveyed. The breakdown according to region was as follows:

North Atlantic	5
South	6
Midwest	4
West	3

In addition to the telephone survey, 15 graduate and undergraduate syllabi were reviewed. These included complete courses in health care policy and strands embedded in other courses.

There was general consensus that integrating health care policy into the nursing curriculum is crucial to the development of nurses as shapers of health care policy and to promotion of autonomous nursing practice and a proactive political involvement on behalf of the nursing profession.

Respondents seemed to agree on the appropriate placement of public policy in the nursing curriculum, based on desired outcomes for each level of education (undergraduate or graduate). At the baccalaureate level, a general awareness of health care policy and politics is expected and in most cases is achieved by including these topics in required upper-division courses, such as community health, issues and trends, and nursing leadership.

At the master's level nursing students are expected to reach a deeper level of understanding. A leadership role is emphasized, so that after graduating these nurses will have the skills and knowledge to be active participants in health care policy.

Expertise in policy analysis and research are the desired outcomes at the doctoral level, with the expectation that these nurses could assume positions in health care policy analysis or research in national, state, or local agencies. Several respondents stressed the need for a systematic approach that links public policy content across each level of nursing education.

Short- and long-term plans for integrating public policy seem to follow a similar pattern. Of those nursing educational programs surveyed, those that have chosen to integrate public policy into the nursing curriculum are planning required or elective graduate-level course in health care policy as their first step. Other short- or long-term plans include establishing institutes or fellowships in health care policy. For instance, the University of Pennsylvania has received a Kellogg Foundation grant to offer an interdisciplinary fellowship in health care policy that includes a summer placement in Washington, D.C. A Division of Nursing grant was awarded to the community health program at the University of Indiana to develop and implement a doctoral program in health care policy.

Several approaches to integrating public policy into nursing curricula are occuring simultaneously. Some nursing education programs are focusing on public policy within their own curricula. At the same time, nurse educators are also looking to expose students to a more interdisciplinary approach by either encouraging them to take courses in other academic departments or including economics or political science faculty in nursing courses. In a few schools, nursing faculty are planning to offer courses in health care policy that will attract students from other disciplines.

Courses in public policy for nursing students were available in several colleges and schools of nursing and also, in almost equal numbers of course offerings, in academic departments outside of the nursing programs. These other departments offering public policy courses are business and health services administration, public affairs, public health, political science, economics, and law.

Faculty had generally positive attitudes toward the importance of public policy in the nursing curriculum. However, the realities of an already full curriculum and scarce resources presented many challenges and, in some cases, obstacles to implementation.

Survey results clearly indicated that there are relatively few faculty members who are well prepared to teach health care policy. Some are doctorally prepared or have extensive experience in the field of health care policy, but they are the exception rather than the rule. Many programs indicated that they lack well-prepared nursing faculty for health care policy and therefore rely on outside guest lecturers.

Educational resources for teaching health care policy to nurses are limited, perhaps because of the relative newness of the topic in the curriculum. Most faculty rely on periodicals and journals, textbooks, government documents, and field trips. The majority of respondents indicated the need for resources such as audiovisual aids, case studies, introduction of public policy content in other nursing texts, and a wider range of scholarly material on health care policy.

Discussion of the Survey Findings

Several major trends emerged from the survey. First, faculty and students appear to be increasingly interested in health care policy and are giving it a higher priority than in the past in terms of curriculum development. However, there is a range of differences in the extent to which these programs integrate public policy into their curricula.

Second, this heightened awareness can be contrasted with the challenges many deans and faculties face in actually making space for public policy in the curriculum. Requiring that master's level nursing students take a course in health care policy (especially if it means eliminating or redesigning other core courses), assigning clinical experiences in place of more traditional clinical practice, and educating faculty to teach or participate in health care policy are some of the more frequently cited issues needing resolution when decisions are made to integrate health care policy into nursing educational programs.

Third, it was clear that overall there is a scarcity of nursing faculty well prepared to teach health care policy on the graduate level. Several schools report offering faculty the opportunity to pursue two-to-four-week internships in federal or state legislative or regulatory agencies. These experiences are mutually beneficial to both the faculty and the agency officers. However, these experiences are not a substitute for the hiring of doctorally prepared faculty in health care policy.

The survey indicated that faculty preparation is an area that warrants as much attention as course content and curriculum development. Developing a cadre of nurse faculty who are doctorally prepared in health policy must occur simultaneously with efforts to integrate policy into course content.

Despite the limited availability of faculty, programs that have developed nursing curricula in health care policy have designed courses and strands which are well-planned, thorough, and include many important and timely issues in health care policy.

REVIEW OF PUBLIC POLICY SYLLABI

Review of available undergraduate and graduate syllabi focused on course titles, objectives, content, methodologies, and reading and reference lists. Strands of courses and specific health policy courses were summarized, combined, and categorized in an effort to identify common themes. A distinction was made between undergraduate and graduate syllabi, with the exception of methodologies. Because some methodologies could apply to both undergraduate and graduate health care policy content, they were combined so that faculty can choose from a larger array of techniques.

The results of this review may be used as a resource for undergraduate and graduate faculty who are developing courses in health care policy. They also form the basis for the model course described later in this chapter. A detailed listing of the results follows.

Undergraduate

Categories of Titles

    Policy/politics of health
    Policy related to specific populations

Health care system
Professional role development/issues

Objectives

1. Identify the sociopolitical issues and problems relevant to nursing and health care.
2. Analyze the factors (socioeconomic, political, historical) that influence the development of nursing and health care public policy.
3. Define and describe the political, legislative, and policy processes.
4. Discuss strategies for influencing nursing health care policy.
5. Participate in political activities (individually and collectively).

Course Content

History of health care
American government: The three branches
The nature of public problems and policy: Policy making and analysis
Political participation: Power, politics, PACs, and professional nursing organizations
Health care services and delivery: Focus on specific populations (chronic illness, elderly, occupational health, MCH) and international issues
Health economics and financing
Women and politics

Graduate

Categories of Titles

Policy
Policy related to clinical focus
Legislation
Politics
Leadership/advanced role development

Objectives

1. Analyze the major problems in the health care delivery system from socioeconomic, political, ethicolegal, technological, and historical perspectives.
2. Analyze major issues, policies, and interrelationships relevant to the nation's health care system from a policy analysis framework.

3. Evaluate theories (e.g., power), ideologies (e.g., distributive justice), and public policy paradigms (e.g., incrementalism).
4. Analyze roles and influences of various participants in policy making, especially nurses as influencers.
5. Synthesize information on the process of health care formulation (including legislation) from concept to development to evaluation, including the role of the nurse in each phase.
6. Propose alternative strategies or solutions to policy-related problems.
7. Develop leadership skills necessary to shape health care policy.

Course Content

Developing health care policy at the federal and state level
Problem identification
Process of government: Legislation and regulation
Policy analysis: Models and techniques
Competition versus regulation in health care
Supply and demand for health care: Manpower and technology
Political economy/health care financing: PPS, third-party reimbursement, Medicare and Medicaid
Quality assurance techniques: PROs
Special issues: MCH, elderly, organ transplants, indigent population
Distributive justice/ethics/legal issues
Cultural, environmental, and mass media influence on policy
Policy evaluation, program evaluation
Policy research
Modes of health care delivery
The health care system: Comparative and international perspectives
Alternative approaches and the future of health care
Political mobilization and participation: Campaigning, the electorate, lobbying, personal politics
Women and politics

Teaching Methods

Lecture, discussion, use of guest speakers
Seminar
Field experiences
	Attend meetings: city council, PACs, nursing associations, hearings
	Meet with legislator

Write legislator
Attend Lobby Day
Visit library for legislative, political, and policy resources
Bring to class definitions of concepts
Case study analysis
Instructional packages (self-instruction)
Oral presentations
   Debate forum
   Group reports on class projects
   Policy updates
   Arguments for policy alternatives
   Group testimony/hearings
Examinations: midterm and final
Written assignments
   Bibliography cards on articles
   Write testimony
   Write a briefing paper
   Write a position paper
   Development and solution of major health care issues
   Manuscript to submit to a journal
   Analyze the legislative history of an issue
   Fact sheet
   Analyze political dimensions (power dynamics) of a real-life
      situation (personal, job, or professional politics)
   Written analysis of cases using general guidelines
   Identify the president's stand on health policies
   List ten national organizations interested in health policy
   Analyze a specific political issue relevant to nursing
   Identify and discuss one issue relevant to women and nursing
   Write a resolution on a health matter for the 1987 NLN con-
      vention
   Analyze a process involved in the passage of a specific piece
      of state nursing or health legislation
   Design a strategy for promoting a specific piece of national
      nursing or health policy
   Summarize legislative history of a bill and its disposition
   Review key political actors and health issues
   Complete a policy analysis, including ethicolegal, social, health,
      political, and economic considerations
   Issue analysis, including issues, players
   Critique of a research study
   Policy proposal with a solution considering cost containment

Books on the reading and reference lists were tabulated for frequency with which they were used and ten "best sellers" were identified. These are listed in Chapter 7. In addition, books that represent some of the classic work in the field of public policy, as well as books and journals and other sources of background reading for faculty and students, are cited in Chapter 7.

Discussion of Syllabi Findings

The review of the syllabi validated the notion that undergraduate education in health care policy is designed to promote awareness, while graduate education promotes in-depth understanding and expertise. For the most part, undergraduate nursing faculty introduced health care policy in required nursing courses. Some faculty used the innovative approach of including health care policy in courses on topics such as chronic illness and health of populations.

The graduate nursing faculty used a variety of approaches, ranging from discussing the legislative process and current policy issues to emphasizing understanding of policy analysis and research. Faculty members who taught health care policy courses in doctoral programs focused exclusively on policy research.

For baccalaureate graduates, exposure to health care policy utilizing strands of content in a variety of clinically focused and role-development courses appears to be appropriate. The scope of practice for master's and doctorally prepared nurses requires more extensive knowledge and skills in applying policy to practice. For doctorally prepared nurses, the greater level of expertise dictates the necessity for more intensive content and requires that space be made in the curriculum for more than one course. Integrating health care policy into the master's curriculum is more complex, because health policy must compete with the many other requirements needed to prepare nursing leaders at this level. In cultivating nursing leaders who are able to participate in today's multifaceted health care environment, it is important that public policy be given equal consideration with other required topics that promote the versatility of the master's prepared nurse. In order to accomplish this, a separate course in health care policy should be offered. The following model health care policy course is presented to assist those nurse faculty who will be responsible for designing such a master's level course.

THE MODEL COURSE

The syllabus for the model course includes course title, overview, objectives, a content outline for 16 weeks or one semester, and teaching methods. The reference list may be developed from the citations found in Chapter 7.

The following guidelines are offered to graduate faculty who are interested in using this model course:

- The course is organized into seven modules, each of which is designated in the content outline by a roman numeral. Each module contains from one to three classes.
- The modules are arranged in a logical sequence for those faculty who opt to use the entire course.
- Each module is self-contained to provide faculty with the flexibility to use any module as a separate lecture or as part of another nursing course.
- The outline for the course is comprehensive and the content is meant to be taught as is. Nevertheless, due to time constraints and individual preferences, faculty may choose to delete certain topics.
- Faculty interested in background reading for content cited in the course outline should refer to Chapter 7.
- Several methods of teaching public policy in the classroom are used in this course. Lecture and seminar discussion provide students with an opportunity to build their knowledge base and to explore the implications of the material. Other techniques, such as the case studies referred to in classes 11 and 12, give students first-hand experience in the process of policy analysis.
- For faculty who wish to use the case study method, Chapter 8 contains a discussion of this method and two case studies, keyed to classes 11 and 12. Suggestions for other case studies are included in the syllabus.
- The case studies are reprinted in the *Student Workbook* that accompanies this book, in addition to a glossary, bibliography, and exercises for students.

Model course

Title

Public Policy and Nursing

Overview

This course provides a foundation for nurses who will participate in all aspects of public policy and for those who strive to be public policy leaders. The focus is on the interrelationships between the policy process, the role of the nurse, and the delivery of health care. Students will analyze health care policy from socioeconomic, ideological, political, and technological perspectives. Students will acquire skills in policy analysis, strategic planning for improving health care policy, and political participation to advance the profession of nursing.

Objectives

At the end of this course participants will be able to:

1. Analyze the major problems in the health care delivery system from socioeconomic, political, ethicolegal, technological, and historical perspectives.
2. Evaluate major issues and policies relevant to the nation's health care system from the perspective of health care policy analysis.
3. Describe theories, ideologies, and paradigms relevant to public policy.
4. Analyze the roles of various participants in policy making, especially nurses as influencers.
5. Synthesize information on health care issues through policy analysis and program evaluation.
6. Develop skills to assume leadership roles that will help advance the profession of nursing in the political and policy arenas.

Content

CLASS 1

A. Introduction, review of course and syllabus

I. *Historical Evolution of the Delivery of Health Care and Nursing*

A. Political ideologies: origins of American political thought (Locke, Hobbes, Rousseau, De Tocqueville, Madison, etc.).
B. Origins of public policy for health care; transfer of health care from private to public domain; early women's movement and the role of nursing.
C. Early twentieth-century federal government initiatives in providing health care; the women's suffrage movement, nursing in hospitals and public health settings.

CLASS 2

D. Post–World War II surge in federally funded health care programs (Hill-Burton, Medicare, and Medicaid); manpower shortage; national health insurance; increased use of nurses as providers of care with prime focus on clinical expertise; Great Society programs.

    E. Efforts to control spiraling health care costs (1970s): Tax Equity and Fiscal Responsibility Act (TEFRA), Professional Standards Review Organizations (PSROs), wage and price freeze, Health Systems Agencies (HSAs); emphasis on cost containment; nurses' expanded role; turf battles and the beginnings of nursing research.

    F. Health care reforms of the 1980s: scarce resources, federalism, prospective payment system (PPS), Peer Review Organizations (PROs), financial retrenchment, conservatism; increased political visibility of women and political sophistication of nurses.

CLASS 3

II. Health Policy Analysis and Program Evaluation

    A. Contemporary political ideologies and policy paradigms as they relate to health policy:

        1. Liberalism, conservatism, Marxism.
        2. Rational choice: fact/value dichotomy.
        3. Values critical approach (vis a vis Rein).
        4. Incrementalism.
        5. Structuralism.

    B. Components of the policy process—an overview:

        1. Policymaking: steps and key players.
        2. Policy analysis: prospective and retrospective assessment of policy.
        3. Policy implementation: political environment, economic variables.
        4. Program evaluation: connecting policy and research.

    C. Policymaking:

        1. Assessing national health priorities.
        2. Legislative process.
        3. Regulatory process.
        4. Judicial process.
        5. Key players: legislators, legislative staff members, committees, interest groups.

CLASS 4

    D. Policy analysis:

        1. Rationale for policy analysis as a decision-making technique.
        2. The role of the analyst.
        3. Models that are relevant to health care.
        4. Applying appropriate methodologies (e.g., goals and means, cost-benefit analysis).

E. Program evaluation:
1. Linkages between policy and research.
2. Agencies responsible for program evaluation.
3. Funding.
4. Public versus private sector: differences in responsibility, accountability, finances, and outcomes.
5. The process of evaluating programs.
6. The usefulness of program evaluation (economic and qualitative value in policy formulation and implementation).
7. Dissemination of program evaluation results and other pertinent information.

CLASS 5
III. Politics and Economics of Health Care Financing
A. Economic principles—definitions:
1. Economics.
2. Gross national product (GNP).
3. Fiscal and monetary policy.
4. Supply and demand.
5. Competition versus regulation.
6. Vertical versus horizontal integration.
B. Federal government structures:
1. Office of Management and Budget (OMB).
2. General Accounting Office (GAO).
3. Congressional Budget Office (CBO).
4. Treasury and Federal Reserve.
5. Health Care Financing Administration (HCFA).
C. Budget process:
1. White House.
2. Congress.
3. Authorizations and appropriations.

CLASS 6
D. Prospective payment system (PPS)—acute care:
1. Historical overview: Medicare trust fund; diagnosis related groups (DRGs) seen as one form of PPS (New Jersey, Yale–New Haven, first-generation DRGs, utilization review); Prospective Payment Assessment Commission (ProPAC); congressionally mandated reports.
2. Mechanics of implementation:
a. From 23 medical diagnosis categories to 468 DRGs:

principal and primary diagnoses, comorbidity, complications.
b. Financing of DRGs.
c. Waivers, exclusions, outliers.
d. Phase-in over several years.
e. Graduate medical education: direct pass through and indirect adjustments.
3. DRGs and nursing:
a. Costing out of nursing services: relative intensity measures (RIMs), other methods.
b. Patient acuity and severity of illness.
c. Shift to the community.
d. Opportunities for nurses.
4. Challenges under PPS:
a. Cost shifting.
b. Unbundling of services.
c. Disproportionate share/uncompensated care.
d. Proliferation of proprietary chains.
e. Quality-of-care issues.

CLASS 7

E. Effects of PPS on long term care:
1. The crisis: demographics, lack of insurance or other funds.
2. Skilled nursing facilities (SNFs), intermediate care facilities (ICFs), domiciliary care; Medicaid, PPS for SNFs, resource utilization groups (RUGs), aftercare.
3. Community health: reimbursement, who pays? Growth of and current issues in home health care; Medicare and home health care; PPS for community health, copayments and coverage.
4. Case management and coordination of care.
5. Case study: long-term financing.

CLASS 8

This three-hour block of time is to be used by students at their discretion to fulfill the field-experience requirement.

CLASS 9

IV. *Alternative Delivery Systems: Issues and Problems*
A. Deficits in the traditional delivery system:
1. Cost and disincentive to contain costs.
2. Inadequate financing mechanisms: Medicaid fraud and abuse, lack of effective quality control, income testing as

criteria, federal/state administrative dilemmas, high first-dollar coverage, little consumer responsibility, lack of controls on spending and coverage.

3. Limited access: evolution of a two-tier system of health care delivery.
4. Equity and distributive justice: Who gets health care, and who pays for it?
5. Focus on illness care.
6. Lack of acceptance of nonphysician providers.
7. Lack of consumer input in defining services.
8. Fragmentation of services: multisite access to care, effects on the system.
9. Lack of comprehensive planning for distribution of services (local, state, federal).
10. Lack of overall planning for manpower distribution.

B. Alternative approaches:
1. Health maintenance organizations (HMOs).
2. Individual practice associations (IPAs).
3. Preferred provider organizations (PPO).
4. Urgent care centers, ambulatory care centers.
5. Specialty centers (dental, eye, etc.).
6. Day surgery.
7. Home care services.
8. Self-care and self-help.
9. Services for the elderly: housing units, day care, community centers.
10. Birthing centers.

CLASS 10

11. Financial incentives and third-party payment:
   a. National health insurance and other legislative approaches.
   b. Long-term-care insurance.
   c. Preferred providers.
   d. Business coalitions and employers' role in controlling costs.
   e. Taxing employer-paid benefits.
   f. Prospective payment.
   g. Higher copayment and deductibles.
   h. Health education and consumerism.
   i. Direct third-party reimbursement for nurses.
12. Greater choice of health care providers:

  a. Nurses: practitioners, midwives, clinical specialists.
  b. Social workers.
  c. Physical therapists.
  d. Dietitians/nutritionists.
  e. Clinical psychologists and counselors.
  f. Osteopaths and naturopaths.
  g. Chiropractors.
  h. Holistic health practitioners.
 13. Vertical integration of services: hospitals offering non-acute care services such as home health and hospice.
 14. Greater competitive spirit: marketing, creativity, and innovation in delivery.

CLASS 11

V. Technological, Legal, and Ethical Dimensions of Health Policy
 A. Linkages between technology, law, and ethics.
 B. Technological dimensions:
  1. Defining technology: human and physical resources.
  2. Growth of technology: required changes in definitions and parameters of health and health care.
  3. Government agencies.
  4. Role of the nurse in planning, implementing, and evaluating technology.
  5. Costing issues: tradeoffs between cost and growth.
  6. Rationing of health care technology.
  7. Technology and research:
   a. Relationship between technology and research.
   b. Establishing priorities.
  8. Case studies:
   a. Food and Drug Administration (FDA): new drugs.
   b. Center for Disease Control (CDC): Autoimmune deficiency syndrome (AIDS).
   c. National Institutes of Health (NIH): organ transplants.
 C. Legal dimensions
  1. Legal foundations:
   a. Cases.
   b. Judicial.
   c. Criminal.
  2. Federal Trade Commission (FTC) and antitrust considerations.
  3. Labor law.
  4. Norms and definitions of professional practice:

    a. Nurse practice acts.

    b. Advanced practice: scope-of-practice legislation, third-party reimbursement, supervisory responsibilities, prescribing and clinical privileges.

  5. Malpractice.

  6. Case study: nurse midwives.

CLASS 12

  7. Issues pertaining to patient care:

    a. Freedom of information, access to information (computers).

    b. Patient rights.

    c. Experimental subjects.

  D. Ethical dimensions:

    1. Principles: normative ethics, utilitarianism, ethical pluralism.

    2. Frameworks for ethical decision making.

    3. The appropriate role of government in lowering morbidity and mortality:

      a. How large a role should the government take in health-related issues?

      b. What is the appropriate mode of taxation for funding of health-related problems (e.g., should luxury taxes be used for health promotion and research)?

      c. To what extent should the government interfere with an individual's health (e.g., use of seat belts, laws to restrict driving while intoxicated)?

    4. The nurse's responsibility in handling ethical issues as they relate to public policy: patient advocacy, civic versus professional accountability.

    5. Case study: Baby Doe, organ transplants.

CLASS 13

VI. *Politics and Political Participation*

  A. History of politics in nursing:

    1. Rationale for its growing importance.

    2. Integration with the nursing process.

    3. Update on nurses in public office.

  B. Politics defined (personal, organizational, professional).

  C. Levels of influence:

    1. Public domain.

    2. Organizational.

        a. Position statements.
        b. Organizational structure.
        c. Inter- and intra-organizational politics.
     3. The grass roots body politic:
        a. Political participation.
        b. Political mobilization.
     4. Personal politics:
        a. Values assessment.
        b. Power and influence strategies.
  D. Spheres of influence:
     1. Press/media.
     2. Political action committees (PACs).
     3. Special-interest groups.
     4. The experts (includes academia).
     5. Legislative professionals.
     6. Financial backers and supporters.
     7. Political parties.
  E. Relationships between federal, state, and local politics.
  F. Special issues in politics:
     1. Patronage.
     2. Party politics.
     3. Dirty deals and compromises.
     4. Old boys' network.

CLASS 14

  G. The role of women in politics:
     1. Gender roles.
     2. Socialization of women.
     3. Socialization of nurses.
  H. Political activities:
     1. Voting and voter registration.
     2. Communicating with legislators, both verbal and written.
     3. Campaigning.
     4. Nurse PACs.
     5. Lobbying.
     6. Legislative phone trees.
     7. Networking.
     8. Coalition building.
     9. Running for office.

CLASS 15

VII. *Future Options*
  A. Health planning

1. Sources, both public and private:
    a. Agencies.
    b. Legislative committees and legislators.
    c. Private sector: organizations and individuals.
2. Establishing priorities.
3. Assessment and health planning development.
4. Implementation: challenges and solution.
B. Strategies for change, focusing on:
    1. The health care system.
    2. The nursing profession.
    3. The individual nurse.
C. The nurse as a change agent in public policy:
    1. Leadership role.
    2. Conflict management and negotiation.
    3. Personal assessment and action plan.

CLASS 16

Selected oral presentations by students.

Methodology and evaluation criteria

1. Lecture and seminar discussion: guest lecturers will be used only when they offer a unique perspective because of their academic or experiential backgrounds.
2. Case studies for selected areas of analysis.
3. Selected students' oral presentations: as a basis for class discussion, faculty will select a certain number of students to present their written policy papers to the class. These presentations will not be incorporated into the students' final grades.
4. Policy strategy cards to be handed in at each class with the exception of classes 1, 8, 12, and 16. Each card is worth 1 percent of the final grade. Students will review journal articles from supplemental readings and submit the following information on a 5 × 8″ index card (legible handwriting is acceptable):
    a. A brief overview of the selected article
    b. Salient facts or concepts
    c. Ways in which these facts or concepts can be applied to the role the student will play in the political arena or policy process.
5. Field experience: the student will select one from the recommended list of field experiences. The time allotted for class 8 is to be used to fulfill this requirement. A written report sum-

marizing the experience and listing the major principles learned is to be submitted on or before class 14. Recommended field experiences:

Attend a political action committee meeting.
Attend a legislative committee hearing or mark-up session.
Attend a city council, town hall, or party precinct meeting.
Attend any public- or private-sector health planning meeting.
Interview a legislator or candidate running for office.
Interview a policy analyst or legislative staff person.
Interview an executive in a nursing or health-related organization regarding his or her involvement with public policy.

6. Policy paper: a 10-to-15-page double-spaced typewritten formal paper on a policy issue randomly selected by the student from a representative list of health care policy topics compiled by the instructor. At the first class session, students select their topic from a receptacle that contains an individual slip of paper for each of the policy topics. The rationale for this is to simulate a real-life situation wherein the policy analyst must often deal with unfamiliar material. The paper will include background information, identification of the problem, the policy goals and objectives, analysis of cost factors and the political and economic environment, alternative strategies, and recommended action. This policy paper is due at class 12.

7. Fact sheet: a one-page typewritten paper using a bulleted format that summarizes the salient points of the student's policy paper. This is due with the policy paper at class 12.

8. Class participation: this includes attendance, promptness, participation in seminar and case study discussions and the contribution of relevant questions and comments. Grading criteria:

Policy paper	40%
Fact sheet	15%
Field experience	18%
Class participation	15%
Policy strategy cards	12%
TOTAL	100%

REFERENCES

Bridgman, M. (1966). In B. Bullough & V. Bullough (Eds.), *Issues in nursing.* New York: Springer.

Ehrenreich, B., & English, D. (1973). *Witches, midwives, and nurses: A history of woman healers.* Westbury, NY: The Feminist Press.

Frank, C. M. (1953). *The historical development of nursing.* Philadelphia: Saunders.

Lagemann, E. C. (1983). *Nursing history: New perspectives, new possibilities.* New York: Teachers College Press.

4

CURRICULUM SURVEY:
HEALTH POLICY CONTENT
IN GRADUATE NURSING PROGRAMS

Barbara H. Dunn, Linda C. Hodges, and Judith B. Collins

INTRODUCTION

Policy making is the process through which decisions are made about the allocation and control of resources in our American economic system. To participate in and to influence that process for health care (to speak our truths to those in power), nurses must link thought to action and planning and analysis to politics (Wildovsky, 1979). The necessary link as well as the substantive bases for our truths can be found by integrating health policy content into nursing curricula (Dunn, 1985; Fagin & Maraldo, 1981).

As Sheila Burke ("Senate Outlook," 1985) so succinctly put it, "I don't think individuals can describe themselves as leaders in nursing unless they have a broad understanding of policy and politics." A consensus in support of Burke's opinion has been developing over the past few years, and there is evidence of greater interest among nurses in policymaking at the international, national, state, local, and institutional levels ("ICN '85," 1985; "Nurses Can Spark," 1985; Joel, 1985; Wieczorek, 1985). This consensus and interest is undoubtedly related to the revolutionary changes we are witnessing in health care

financing and delivery. But are these changes reflected in nursing curricula?

CURRICULUM SURVEY

In the fall of 1984, we were involved in developing and teaching
graduate-level courses in health policy for our respective schools of
nursing. As a result, we became interested in the availability and content of similar courses at other schools of nursing. Because this information was not available from a central source, we undertook a survey
research project to collect curriculum data. This chapter reports the
results of that research project.

The research involved a survey of 129 graduate programs in
nursing (N = 127) and public health (N = 2) that are accredited by
the National League for Nursing (NLN, 1984). The programs were
located in 42 states, the District of Columbia, and Puerto Rico: 30 in
the northeast region, 36 in the southeast, 33 in the midwest, 13 in the
southwest, and 16 in the western United States.

In June 1985, a 15-item questionnaire was mailed to graduate
program directors, requesting background data about the programs
as well as information about health policy content in the curriculum.
Major questions that the survey sought to answer were: (1) Is health
policy a substantive area of study in graduate nursing curricula? (2)
How is health policy content integrated into the curriculum? (3) What
factors determine whether a school offers a separate course in health
policy or integrates content into existing courses?

Background Data

Of 129 programs mailed questionnaires, 72 surveys were
returned—a response rate of 56 percent. Responding programs were
located in 34 states and the District of Columbia, with the response
rate higher in the midwest (64%) than in the other regions (southeast,
58%; west, 50%; southwest, 46%; northeast, 43%). These programs
were found in 70 schools of nursing and 2 schools of public health,
a majority of which (68%) were public, state-supported institutions.

While all 72 schools had graduate programs, 56 had only master's
programs and 16 had both master's and doctoral programs. An average of 98 full-time-equivalent students were enrolled in the programs

(range 6–800), which typically had 36 full-time-equivalent faculty members (range 2–160). The major areas of concentration in the curricula were maternal-child health (N = 51), adult medical-surgical (N = 48), nursing administration (N = 39), community health (N = 38), mental health/psychiatric (N = 36), primary care (N = 22), and other subspecialty areas (N = 42) such as oncology, gerontology, and occupational health.

Health Policy Courses

The remainder of the survey responses were related to health policy content. Program directors were asked whether their schools have a required health policy course in the graduate curriculum or whether such a course was available or suggested as an elective. A total of 49 programs had either a required or elective course: 22 programs required and 37 elective (10 programs with required courses also had elective courses). Overall then, 31 percent of respondent programs required this content and 52 percent had a suggested or available elective.

As Table 1 indicates, there were differences in type of course offerings according to program level: that is, whether the school also had a doctoral program. The 16 schools that had both master's and doctoral programs were more likely to have an elective health policy course (10 out of 16, or 62%) than the 56 schools without doctoral programs (27 out of 56; 48%). This difference was not, however, statistically significant. On the other hand, there were no differences with regard to required courses: 30 percent of schools with master's programs only and 31 percent with both master's and doctoral programs offered such courses.

Table 1. Health policy course offering by type of nursing program

| | Type of program | | | | | |
| | Master's | | Master's and doctoral | | All | |
Type of offering	N	%	N	%	N	%
Required and elective	7	12	3	19	10	14
Required only	10	18	2	12	12	17
Elective only	20	36	7	44	27	37
None	19	34	4	25	23	32
TOTAL	56	78	16	22	72	100

The nursing majors in which a health policy course was most frequently required were nursing administration (N = 14) and community health (N = 13). It was more commonly an elective course for students whose areas of concentration were maternal-child health, adult medical-surgical, mental health/psychiatric, and primary care.

There were also regional differences in the frequency of required or elective courses. The highest proportion of programs with required or elective courses were in the northeast (29%) and southeast (29%), followed by the midwest (26%), the western region (10%), and the southwest (6%). On a state-by-state basis, these courses were most likely to be found in the District of Columbia, California, Illinois, and New York.

To summarize, there were differences in course requirements among schools related to nursing majors and geographic location. There were no significant differences according to degree programs available, type of funding (private versus public), or size of the school (as measured by number of faculty members and students). Finally, the number of faculty members prepared to teach this content was not a significant factor in determining whether a course was offered. Teaching responsibility is the subject of the next section.

TEACHING RESPONSIBILITY

Of 49 schools with a required or elective health policy course (a total of 59 courses), 45 courses (76%) carried a nursing course number: 21 out of 22 required courses (one course offered by the school of social work) and 24 out of 37 elective courses. Another 13 elective courses were offered by other schools or departments: public health (N = 4), health administration (N = 4), public administration (N = 2), management/business (N = 2), and social work (N = 1).

These courses were generally taught by a nurse faculty member (33 out of 49 schools, or 67%). Non-nurse faculty members, in the disciplines noted above, taught in another 15 programs (31%), and someone from the community taught at the final program (1 out of 49; 2%).

When program directors were asked how many of their nurse faculty members were prepared to teach health policy content, answers ranged from none (3 programs) to 28 (all faculty members in 1 program). The typical program indicated that there were 3 faculty members prepared, by virtue of education (N = 42), professional involvement

(N = 33), or employment experience (N = 31). An additional 7 responses listed continuing education courses as a method of preparation and 3 indicated that teaching experience was sufficient to prepare their faculty in this area.

Almost one-third of respondents who listed education as a means of preparation to teach health policy indicated nonspecific doctoral education as a qualification. About one-half of those citing education as a qualification specified that the doctoral or master's degrees were in particular content areas (health policy, public health, administration, sociology). Preparation related to professional involvement usually included nursing organizational activities, legislative and lobbying experience, or membership on policy-making bodies. Employment experience (other than teaching) listed most commonly was an administrative position, particularly in a public agency.

In summary, graduate programs with required or elective health policy courses characteristically have a nurse faculty member teach the course, which is usually offered by the school of nursing. One question that arises in analyzing these data is why there is such a discrepancy between the number of faculty members who program directors indicate are prepared to teach this content (average of 3 per program) and the proportion of programs (53%) that either have no course offering (23 out of 72; 32%) or have the course taught by someone other than a nurse faculty member (16 out of 49; 33%).

COURSE CONTENT

Program directors were asked to describe the topical areas covered in their required or elective health policy courses. To facilitate responses, a listing of 45 possible topics was included with the questionnaire. (Provision was also made for additional topics not found in the listing.)

As Table 2 indicates, the topics most frequently cited by respondents (from the listing) were health policy defined, health decision making and the political structure, policy versus politics, and health care financing. These topics were included in an average of 70 percent of the courses. The least popular topics (included in an average of 33 percent of courses) were models of policy analysis, methods and techniques of analysis, and qualitative versus quantitative methods.

In looking at the top 10 and bottom 10 topics, there are some interesting categorical differences. That is, the topics most frequently

Table 2. **Content list: Topics cited in required and elective health policy courses by frequency of citation and rank order**

Topic name and frequency	Rank order
1. Health policy defined (35)	1
2. Health decision making and the political structure (34)	2
3. Policy versus politics (34)	2
4. Health care financing (34)	2
5. Congressional process and health policy (32)	3
6. States' roles in health policy (32)	3
7. Types of policies (31)	4
8. Power: the fundamental concept (31)	4
9. Changing roles of consumers, providers, government, and business (31)	4
10. Politics: the allocation of scarce resources (30)	5
11. Agents of power (30)	5
12. Political savvy—survival tips (30)	5
13. Lobbyists and lobbying: nursing's effectiveness (29)	6
14. Social roles and responsibilities of government and citizens (29)	6
15. Historical review of U.S. health policies and programs (29)	6
16. Trends in organization and financing of health care (29)	6
17. Issues in nursing practice (28)	7
18. Competition versus regulation of health care (28)	7
19. Implementation: rules and regulations, planning, laws (28)	7
20. Participation in policy processes (28)	7
21. State/local political structure (27)	8
22. Political economy of health services (27)	8
23. Regulation/credentialing of services and providers (27)	8
24. Projections related to supply, demand, and future of health care (27)	8
25. Policy processes: formulation, implementation, evaluation (26)	9
26. Roles of government branches (26)	9
27. Values and assumptions underlying policies (25)	10
28. Why study policy making (25)	10
29. Key federal agencies (25)	10
30. Rationing health care services (24)	11
31. Health planning efforts (24)	11
32. Policy spheres, traditional boundaries (23)	12
33. Economic structure/system and policy (23)	12

Table 2. (*Continued*)

Topic name and frequency	Rank order
34. Political participation: women and politics (23)	12
35. Alternative providers and systems of care (22)	13
36. New players: entrepreneurs and corporate interests (22)	13
37. Policy analysis and research (22)	13
38. Competition among providers (21)	14
39. Economic assumptions in market systems (21)	14
40. Rights and privileges in a democratic society (20)	15
41. World health systems: comparative policies (20)	15
42. Distributive justice: the ethics of cost containment (20)	15
43. Models of policy analysis (17)	16
44. Methods/techniques of analysis (16)	17
45. Qualitative versus quantitative methods (15)	18

covered more often relate to political process than to structural or system concerns, specific contemporary issues, or policy analysis and research. On the other hand, the topics covered least frequently cluster in the areas of specific contemporary issues and policy analysis and research.

Integrated Classes

There were also differences in topics covered when health policy content was integrated into existing courses rather than offered in a separate required or elective course. Many programs that do have required or elective courses also integrate content related to health policy into existing courses. Of those survey respondents without a separate course offering (N = 23), only 2 (9%) stated that the content was *not* integrated into other courses. This content was typically integrated into courses in professional issues, leadership and administration, or community health and epidemiology. The average number of hours for the integrated content in health policy was estimated at 7 (range 1–40).

Program directors were asked to indicate (from the topic listing provided) which topic areas were most often included when health policy classes were integrated into other courses. The most common topics were issues in nursing practice and health care financing (67% of responses), followed by the fundamental concept of power and the changing roles of consumers, providers, government, and business (55% of responses). Policy analysis and research, models of policy analysis, methods and techniques of analysis, and implementation of rules and regulations, planning, and laws (5% of responses) were the least popular topics.

Rather than clustering in the political process category, which was the case with the separate courses, the topics covered in integrated classes tended to cluster around specific contemporary issues. Like the separate courses, however, the least popular topics were usually in the policy analysis and research category; several in the bottom 10 clustered in the structural/system concerns group. These findings are not particularly surprising, given the usual structure of professional issues and leadership and administration courses.

PERCEIVED IMPORTANCE OF HEALTH POLICY

A final question was asked of the program directors: On a scale of 1 (not needed) to 8 (crucial), how important is health policy content for graduate nursing curricula? The average answer was 7, indicating that respondents believe this content to be very important. The importance attributed to the content, however, was not a statistically significant factor in determining whether a school offered a required or elective course to teach this content. This and other survey findings answer some questions and raise others.

If these results are indicative of graduate nursing curricula in general, the answer to the question, Is health policy a substantive area of study in graduate nursing curricula? is unequivocally *no*. More than two-thirds (69%) of the programs responding to the survey do not require a formal course in this content area. Although 51 percent of programs have a suggested or available elective, one-third of these courses are offered in another department or school. Among those programs without a separate course, an average of only 7 hours of content related to health policy is integrated into other courses.

How is health policy content integrated into graduate nursing curricula? These results suggest that it is most often offered as an elective course rather than as a curriculum requirement. If it is required, nursing administration and community health majors are the graduate students most likely to have such a requirement. Existing courses in professional issues, leadership and administration, and community health and epidemiology are those in which health policy classes are usually integrated.

What factors determine whether a school offers a separate course in health policy or integrates content into existing courses? The answer to this question is unclear. The decision does not appear to be related to the importance attributed to this content, the number of faculty members prepared to teach the content, presence of a doctoral program, program funding, or program size. It does appear to be related to geographic differences that seem consistent with centers of regional political activity and state-level political involvement among nurses.

Some of the questions that this research raises include the following. (1) If health policy content is crucial for graduate nursing curricula, why do so few programs offer a required course? (2) For the small proportion of schools with a required course, why is this content deemed more essential for some majors than others? (3) If there are an average of 3 nurse faculty members per program prepared to teach this content, why are one-third of the courses that are available taught by a non-nurse faculty member in another school or department or by someone from outside the institution? (4) Can it be said that nurse faculty members are qualified to teach this content by virtue of non-specific doctoral education or teaching experience or involvement in professional organizations? (5) Why do existing courses seem to emphasize political variables in the policy-making process, rather than providing equal emphasis for the rational variables (knowledge and organization)? (Doty, 1980).

SUMMARY DISCUSSION

Like Burke ("Senate Outlook," 1985), we believe that leaders and leadership in nursing require a broad understanding of policy and politics. Without this understanding, our knowledge of decision making may be parsimonious and our perspective on the world parochial (Joel, 1985). It is precisely that lack of knowledge and perspective that has contributed, historically, to the absence of effective leadership in nursing and other women's occupational groups.

The development of leadership skills in *all* master's students is a characteristic of graduate education in nursing, according to the National League for Nursing. How do graduate schools of nursing define leadership, if not in relation to policy making, and how are these skills and knowledge addressed in the curriculum? If health policy course requirements are primarily targeted at graduate students in nursing administration and community health, where do clinicians obtain this information? Can we expect to bridge the practice–policy gap without this knowledge base among master's prepared clinicians? In regard to doctoral programs without health policy course requirements, how can we prepare scholars, researchers, educators, or clinical leaders without providing them with grounding related to the rational and political variables that influence decision making?

This research indicates that there is incongruence between graduate educators' philosophy about the importance of health policy content and their practice in integrating that content into the curriculum. In addition, we believe that program directors have overestimated the number of faculty members prepared to teach this content. The estimates of faculty preparation seem to place substantial emphasis on experiential learning and nonspecific education. If we believe that this type of preparation is adequate to qualify a faculty member to teach health policy, we must deny that there is a body of disciplinary knowledge specific to health policy and policy making that requires theoretical as well as experiential understanding.

In summary, our stage of development in relation to health policy content in graduate nursing curricula is roughly equivalent to where we were with health assessment 10 years ago. And, as with health assessment, we expect that faculty comfort and effectiveness in teaching this content can be increased by participation in intensive, short-term faculty development courses and that learning (for both students and faculty) is facilitated by courses that provide for didactic presentations and a policy making practicum. In another 10 years, past experience with health assessment may become prologue: health policy will be core content in graduate nursing programs and in undergraduate programs as well. The findings of this survey demonstrate that graduate nursing programs have just begun to address the issue of integrating health policy content into the curriculum. We will continue to monitor their progress.

REFERENCES

Doty, P. (1980). *Guided change of the American health system— Where the levers are.* New York: Human Sciences Press.

Dunn, B. H. (1985). Speaking truth to power. *Nursing Economics, 3*, 8.

Fagin, C., & Maraldo, P. (1981). *Health policy in the nursing curriculum: Why it's needed.* New York: National League for Nursing.

ICN '85. (1985). *American Journal of Nursing, 85*, 918.

Joel, L. A. (March–April 1985). Nurses as policymakers: An analysis of the dynamics of power. *Orthopaedic Nursing, 4*, 6.

National League for Nursing. (1984). *Master's education in nursing: Route to opportunities in contemporary nursing, 1984–85.* New York: NLN.

Nurses can spark social change, say ICN speakers. (July–August 1985). *The American Nurse, 17*, 19.

Senate outlook: An interview with Sheila Burke. (1985). *Nursing & Health Care, 6*, 249.

Wieczorek, R. R. (Ed.). (1985). *Power, Politics and Policy in Nursing.* New York: Springer.

Wildavsky, A. (1979). *Speaking truth to power: The art and craft of policy analysis.* Boston: Little, Brown.

5

TEACHING PUBLIC POLICY

Sister Rosemary Donley

This chapter considers some dimensions of teaching public policy. Some of the issues are internal to the work of the faculty. These include the merits of integrating public policy into the curriculum, curriculum development, and the placement of policy courses or content within the program of study. The second part of the discussion will consider course content, methods of teaching, and selection of field sites. These issues are generic to any discussion of curriculum change. However, the nature of the text prompts me to analyze curriculum change as a political process rather than an educational one.

CURRICULAR ISSUES

Consensus about the role of the nurse is critical to the development of a curriculum (O'Rourke, 1981). If the faculty decides that the nurse is a teacher of patients, the program of study will look different from a curriculum planned to prepare bedside nurses. Curricula that

The author acknowledges the sensitive reading and advice given by Myra Snyder, PhD, executive director, California Nurses' Association.

prepare nurses for policy making reflect this orientation in electives, core courses, and field experiences. Successful introduction of public policy into the curriculum requires acknowledgement that the scope of professional practice includes policy making. Convincing colleagues that policy making is integral to professional nursing practice requires a strategy similar to lobbying. Several models of influence can be used. Most schools of nursing teach undergraduate courses in trends and issues. These usually include discussions about legal aspects of practice (practice acts), health care financing (reimbursement), and political action. Small changes (incremental change) can be introduced into these courses by showing the relationships between law making and policy development. For example, efforts to amend nurse or medical practice acts are usually motivated by economic policy. Nursing associations seek bills that will enable nurses to enlarge their domains of work and remove the concept of medical supervision from their practice acts. Medical associations block nurses in their efforts to change the language of practice acts to ensure medical autonomy and income protection. Students can be helped to see that their practice acts not only define nursing but also provide the foundation for scope of work, autonomy, and income (Aydelotte, 1983). In other words, law dictates policy.

The legislative struggles to amend practice acts are often taught under the rubrics of professionalism, nursing theory, or standards of practice. It is possible, however, to discuss practice acts using such health policy concepts as need, access, distribution, and reimbursement. The use of a policy framework connects practice to the public's need for care. Regulation of practice by the state introduces standards more oriented to consumer protection than professional dominance. In states where there are mandatory practice acts, professional credentials are given to those who meet statutory requirements. Several years ago, when the Rural Health Clinics Act was established by federal law, reimbursement for nurses was linked to recognition of expanded practice in state practice acts. Use of policy concepts in teaching about practice acts balances the tendency to teach the practice of nursing according to professional themes. Even if faculty members are ambivalent about the role of the nurse as policy maker, health policy frameworks provide another mode of understanding the complicated relationships between law and behavior. This idea can be emphasized in lobbying faculty colleagues.

Examining the process of amending or protecting practice acts also provides an occasion to illustrate politically motivated behavior. Political action is directed toward attaining power and controlling the allocation of resources. Political bias expresses the value system of interest groups. In the United States, political behavior is ascribed to elected officials. However, professional groups operate from political as well as ideological and professional motivation. Legislative actions can be analyzed from the viewpoint of special interest groups. For example, professional nursing associations seek to strengthen the legal position of nurses and to give nurses control over the implementation of their practice acts. This behavior is rationalized as professional and normative. Nurses argue that they are most knowledgeable about their own practice and are therefore best able to set educational criteria, establish practice standards, and discipline and control the practice of professional peers. Because most nurses have been socialized into this view, it may be startling to label activism in regard to practice acts as an illustration of political special interest. Nurses who enter the political arena of practice legislation with ideological stances and theoretical positions are quickly disillusioned. The classroom can provide a forum to look at practice acts from multiple perspectives.

Perhaps the desire to preserve professional integrity is the best argument for the introduction of public policy into the curriculum. If the Social Policy Statement of the American Nurses' Association is correct, nurses fulfill a social mandate (ANA, 1980). However, social mandates cannot exist in isolation from society. Teaching professional nursing as part of a policy agenda enables students to see how public and societal wishes are integral to professional behavior. Public policy places parochial and professional concerns about practice within a decisional framework in which the common good, safety of clients and protection of patients, becomes the criteria for selection of a course of action.

The methods that have been suggested to introduce health policy into traditional curricula have included expansion of agenda (enlarging the definition of practice), incrementalism (adding to existing concepts or rationales), and appealing to previously held positions and policies (reinterpreting professionalism to include a social mandate.) Practice acts were chosen as the vehicle for change because they are a common theme in curricula.

Graduate Curricula

It is easy to discuss curriculum patterns in undergraduate programs. However, graduate education is specialized and more heterogeneous. Graduate programs may include courses in trends, health care delivery, and professional roles. If these courses exist, the strategies suggested to modify the undergraduate curriculum are appropriate. If the graduate program lacks a curriculum structure compatible with the addition of health policy, new modules or courses must be introduced. Adding to the curriculum agenda requires negotiation and compromise. Faculty colleagues must be persuaded to review content and time of instruction. If there are no benefits or trade-offs, faculty members may be unwilling to change their patterns or give up vested interests. Because a curriculum change represents a new agenda, it becomes important to understand the values, attitudes, and bases of power of those who control it. If a seniority system is operative within the faculty organization, junior members have little opportunity to change the curriculum unless they can enlist their senior colleagues and convince the most influential among them of the merit of their ideas. This goal can be brought into reach of junior members who can win the trust of their senior colleagues. This may mean that junior faculty members patiently place their ideas on the curriculum committee's agenda and work to reduce ambiguity and unfamiliarity. Another strategy is to seize the opportunity of curriculum evaluations, revision, or accreditation and change the agenda. In this scenario, the faculty is viewed as a congressional committee in which junior members must "wait their turns," establish their credibility, win the support of senior colleagues, or change the rules before their ideas (bills) will be seriously considered. In any discussion of the curriculum, it is important to remember that the curricular agenda represents the history, hopes, aspirations, and vested interests of the senior faculty. The curriculum is an important policy document because it contains the decisions about what is important (issues), methods of addressing the issues (technologies), values (norms), and roles (implementations). Consequently, senior faculty members, who usually teach graduate courses, are likely to resist change. In the political world, seasoned lobbyists would plan carefully before attempting to influence such a group.

Most texts in curriculum development discuss ideal placement of content to assist students in the logical development of their ideas. However, unless faculty members are responsive to the introduction of public policy into the curriculum, discussions about the ideal placement of concepts are interesting but nonproductive. While there may be a best place to insert policy ideas, modules can be appended to any course, just as amendments can be attached to any bill or law. At the end of legislative sessions, when logic overshadows politics, congressional staffs sort out and integrate amendments into appropriate legislative categories. Some faculties spend a session every few years reviewing the placement of material, rearranging, and fine tuning the curriculum. Some attention should be given to the evolution of a curriculum process that separates the acceptance of new ideas from the placement of these ideas within the established curriculum.

An interesting political lesson about compromise can be learned during curriculum committee meetings. If a group has invested time and energy in a particular rationale, they may be unwilling to see it examined and modified. When faculty members identify intellectually or emotionally with curriculum rationales, they find compromise and negotiation demeaning and dissonant to their beliefs. Some advocates of change feel discouraged and defeated if their proposals are modified. However, an idea or program rarely moves forward without modification by the approving bodies. When the faculty reaches such an impasse in its discussions, it becomes important to differentiate goals and means. One approach is to seek common agreement on principles. It is possible to strategize so that everyone wins a little and no one loses everything. This approach may not satisfy the zealots, but it enables the group to go forward after decisions are made.

Setting agendas is another key concept in public policy. Any agenda—the curriculum is a good example—represents a constellation of important issues. Each issues has its own constituency. Changing the agenda (adding to, deleting from) shifts the bases of power. It is an unusual group that abdicates power (Donley, 1983). Because faculty are keepers of the tradition (the curriculum), they must be informed and influenced to believe that change will enrich their programs of study and their personal power. Part of this reorientation is intellectual. Experts can be invited to discuss public policy theory, health policy issues, and political strategies (agenda setting, issue formulation, lobbying, the legislative and regulatory process) with the faculty. The panel of experts that is assembled should reflect theoretical and practical concerns and represent opinions about local, regional, and national issues. While the financing of this educative process may seem to be prohibitive, it requires more planning than money. Political science faculty can usually be encouraged to give lectures on policy and political theory. Spokespersons from health or professional lobbies or organizations are always willing to lay out the issues of their groups. The staff members of state legislators and those who work in district offices of representatives and senators can add another perspective by explaining their work with constituents. The more representative the panel of experts, the broader the spectrum of issues that can be identified. Discussion should elicit the way in which each group deals with issue analysis and management and develops political strategies. During the seminars, faculty will see that political processes intersect policy

processes at many stages of formulation and implementation. However, while policy development can be explained in seminars, introduction to the political process requires immersion in a political campaign
or involvement in grass-roots political action.

The model of faculty continuing education presented here has its
parallel in government. Members of Congress or legislators hold hearings to learn about issues or bring about consensus. During the hearing,
experts are invited to present testimonies of fact, theory, and opinion.
Occasionally legislators make site visits to investigate problem areas
or observe models of the programs under examination. The program
of faculty development that has been outlined is similar to a hearing.
If hearings (faculty educational programs) have been successful, decision makers bring information and experience to the task at hand.
Hearings also enable members of Congress and their staffs to identify
the agendas of special-interest groups and to determine support for
the issue that prompted the hearing. During faculty discussions, attitudes about public policy can be explored, power brokers can be
identified and involved in the change process, vested interests about
the curriculum can be brought into the open, and resources can be
assessed. When the curriculum is examined to determine if it will be
changed, the faculty is in better position to negotiate and compromise.

The last issue of curriculum development that will be discussed
is the merit of integrating policy concepts into several courses. I believe
it is better to teach a separate course than to integrate public policy
into many courses. Integration requires high levels of commitment to
the process, as well as a great deal of planning and oversight. The
involvement of several faculty members requires continuous orientation and frequent meetings. Overlap, repetition, and the tendency to
address the same concepts in each course are difficult problems to
overcome.

After the faculty has agreed to introduce public policy into the
curriculum, it begins the interesting task of selecting course content
(Fagin & Maraldo, 1981). Students should study some political theory,
policy process, and selected health issues. The political theory may
include an overview of American government (the legislative and regulatory systems), agenda setting, and policy development, implementation, and evaluation. Process modules teach law making, group
dynamics, lobbying, negotiation, management of conflict, and consensus building. While it is easy to lay out policy and process content, it
is more difficult to reach agreement about health issues. This task is
simplified by decisions about the inclusion of national or local issues.
Faculty should select or enable students to choose issues from a na-

tional, regional, or local perspective. Faculty and students can also be guided in their selection of issues by sampling policy categories. Historically, health services, manpower, health financing, and research and development have been useful organizational constructs at the national level. If faculty and students opt for a national agenda, a sampling of national issues might resemble this pattern: Community Nursing Centers (health services), Nursing Training Act (manpower) prospective payment and DRGs (financing), and National Institute of Nursing (research and development).

Another way of identifying issues to be studied is to examine the most important issues of various constituents. This approach was illustrated in the faculty continuing education program, where multiple special-interest groups were asked to present their major health issue. Examining the regulatory process and its impact on policy illustrates another design for a course. Regulatory activity to protect human subjects or legislation to ensure access to care for high-risk handicapped newborns, the so-called Baby Doe legislation, shows how public issues also involve providers and institutions. Issues that address the implementation and regulation of public policy open up a new literature, spawn new constituents, and challenge faculty and students to think creatively about nursing roles in public policy.

Another way of selecting course content is to use the policy process itself (issue identification, development, formulation, legislation, implementation and evaluation) as a framework for tracking issues. This process approach to teaching policy is analogous to the longitudinal and cross-sectional sampling familiar in clinical education. Faculty who teach maternal-child health nursing by assigning students to childbearing families for long-term study and to parents in various stages of pregnancy, labor, and postpartal experience will be familiar with this pedagogical technique. Faculty and students may find that their longitudinal tracking of an issue may be carried out in one semester. However, legislative processes are like soap operas: students usually build on and enrich the work of their peers in previous semesters as they develop their own portfolios.

TEACHING STRATEGIES

Most teaching strategies to be selected are not unique to the teaching of public policy. These are some differences. While there are several videotapes on health issues available for purchase, significant audiovisual holdings are yet to be developed. In my teaching, I have found that assigning students real-world tasks is informative and gives them experience in using policy concepts. Students develop briefing papers that explain in one page the salient concepts and political overtones of proposed bills or amendments. One-page assignments can also challenge students to synthesize or differentiate among various amendments or bills, abstract hearings, or analyze positions of special-interest groups. More sophisticated assignments invite students to develop a historical analysis of a particular bill or law, propose a policy model for a hearing, or develop option papers in which they identify and test the consequences of alternative policy options. Evaluative standards emphasize conciseness, realism, practicality, and creativity in evolving policy options.

If the faculty opts to include a practicum with the course, it can select among executive, legislative, and regulatory agencies or special or public interest groups. The location of the nursing program may be a major factor in selecting sites (Cowart, 1981). Certainly schools located in major or capital cities are well positioned to select for student experience. More significant than the identification of places is a consideration of expectations to be achieved from the experience. One obvious outcome is that students will learn the work of the agency and how it conducts its business. These insights are helpful if the nurses are to engage in policy formation. Faculty and students also learn something about the relationship of objectives to the political or policy process. The a priori writing of objectives is designed to exert some measure of control and structure. However, students lack the ability to exert influence on district congressional offices, professional organizations, or special interest groups. Students or their teachers do not set the agenda. While students work faithfully on achieving prescribed objectives, they may miss opportunities to observe or participate in policy-oriented behavior or political action. One technique that can be used to encourage students to seek unpredictable experiences is to write a broad objective, such as to describe and analyze at least one unplanned political or policy experience with each session. This objective will encourage students to poke around the offices and listen to the grapevine. Faculty can use students' logs as a tool in supervision and evaluation. Political offices resemble labor-and-delivery suites or emergency rooms in city hospitals, in that a great deal is always going on, often behind the scenes, and decisions are made rapidly. One of the challenges is to learn how to shift priorities without losing sight of major objectives. Students should be encouraged to explore with their mentors and colleagues in the field the values and goals that drive the offices. This exercise may prove to be enlightening and seminal to their introduction into public policy.

Who will teach public policy? I believe that if the faculty is committed to the end, it will find the means. Some schools of nursing now offer policy courses or special policy tracks as part of the curriculum. Most political science departments teach courses in American government. Some teach public policy as a specialized field. Several organizations, such as the Institute of Medicine, offer competitive fellowships (Zwick, 1982; see also Chapter 7 of this book). Nurses have been selected for these awards. The National League for Nursing, the American Nurses' Association, and the Federation of Specialty Nursing Associations sponsor policy workshops and help negotiate field assignments. The Washington Round Table was organized in 1980 as an informal network for nurses interested in policy. Every health organization publishes legislative newsletters and information sheets (see Chapter 7). Health policy is a category in the *Cumulative Index Medicus*, the National Library of Medicine current catalog, and the *International Nursing Review*. Federal and state governments print bills, laws, regulatory documents, and reports of hearings. While the resources to teach public policy may be harder to find than clinical texts, they exist in each community.

Early nurse authors encouraged nurses to be citizens. After suffrage was achieved, this statement seemed to lose its meaning. Today there is a new interest in public life and the field of public policy is a new arena for nurses. As the cost of care becomes the major issue in health, attention to the policy process will stimulate nurses to conduct research on cost-effective strategies of care. The importance of this knowledge and the need for nurses to contribute to the interdisciplinary field of health services research is the best argument for the inclusion of public policy in nursing education.

REFERENCES

American Nurses' Association. (1980). *Nursing: A social mandate.* Kansas City, MO: American Nurses' Association.

Aydelotte, M. (1983). Professional nursing: The drive for governance. In N. Chaska (Ed.), *The nursing profession: A time to speak.* New York: McGraw-Hill.

Cowart, M. (1981). *Implementing health policy in baccalaureate nursing curricula.* New York: National League for Nursing.

Donley, Sr. R. (1983). Nursing and the politics of health. In N. Chaska (Ed.), *The nursing profession: A time to speak.* New York: McGraw-Hill.

Fagin, C., & Maraldo, P. (1981). *Health policy in the nursing curriculum: Why it's needed.* New York: National League for Nursing.

O'Rourke, M. (1981). *Health policy: The clinical perspective.* New York: National League for Nursing.

Zwick, D. (1982). Evaluation of the Robert Wood Johnson Health Policy Fellowship program: A synopsis. *Journal of Health Politics, Policy and Law, 6,* 780–782.

6

HEALTH SERVICES RESEARCH
AND THE FORMULATION OF PUBLIC POLICY

Jeffrey C. Merrill, Marcia M. Sass, and Stephen A. Somers

INTRODUCTION

Is health services research important in the formulation of public policy? There are some who would argue that such research is critical to the development of public policy; others contend that policy makers seldom rely on, or are even aware of, relevant reasearch. Good research, however, does not necessarily lead to sound policy.

There is truth in what both groups contend: a gap does exist between the policy maker and the researcher. Bridging that gap is important, both to strengthen the decision-making process and to justify continued or expanded support for health services research. There is a great deal of talk about research, specifically nursing research, and public policy. This chapter explains the linkage between the two and what must be done to strengthen it.

In attempting to bridge this gap, it would be helpful to describe what is meant by health services research. Health services research focuses on the organization, distribution, and delivery of health services. The financing of health care, manpower, quality of care, cost–benefit analysis of various programs, and the feasibility of delivering care in alternative settings are some of the issues encompassed. Program evaluation is a major thrust of health services research.

Health policy research is health services research that is conducted and used for addressing aspects of health policy at the local, state, or national level. It tends to be outcome oriented; cost–benefit/effectiveness and patient outcomes are the key elements studied. Given this brief background, there are three basic categories of health services research that can be used for the development of health policy:

1. Descriptive research, or the reporting and analyzing of data on what exists: mortality rates, levels of health insurance, utilization of specific services, the distribution of nurse midwives. Such efforts might entail the collection of primary data or the analysis of existing secondary data sources.

It should be noted that although descriptive research may appear to be policy neutral, its effect can be very much a function of how it is presented. For example, recent data on a continuing decline in infant mortality rates (cup half full) were reported in a way that emphasized that the *rate* of decline had slowed (cup half empty). While this concern over abatement in the rate of decline is justified, it does demonstrate how the same data can be used in opposite ways to evoke different public or political responses.

2. Demonstration projects are limited efforts to determine the effectiveness of a specific program or intervention before expanding such efforts to a broader population. Demonstrations, by definition, include an evaluation as an integral component of their development. The majority use quasi-experimental designs, meaning that similar groups that do not receive an intervention and are not under the investigator's control are selected and compared with the experimental or intervention group. Some demonstrations are randomized clinical trials (RCTs), which are designed as true experiments. In RCTs, both the intervention and comparison groups are under the investigator's control. Examples of demonstrations important to nursing include the recently completed hospice demonstration, which was a limited effort, in 26 sites, intended to evaluate whether this form of care for terminally ill patients should be covered under Medicare. Also, the National Teaching Nursing Home Program was intended to demonstrate whether upgrading geriatric nursing training would lead to improvements in patient functional status, lower costs of care, and fewer hospitalizations.

While many demonstrations involve multiple sites, others are limited to a single site. For example, the Health Care Financing Administration (HCFA) has just awarded funds to the Kaiser/Portland HMO to test the effectiveness of some interventions intended to reduce the incidence of falls among the elderly at that one site.

3. Retrospective evaluations are analyses of programs already in place, such as the Women's, Infants', and Children's Food and Nutrition Program (WIC) or the Head Start program. Such evaluations assess the effects of existing programs to determine whether they should be continued. Evaluating a program already in place is likely to be difficult, however, since that program was probably developed with little or no thought to the feasibility of ultimately evaluating it. In a demonstration, a control group might have been identified as part of the planning of the project. However, for an already widely implemented program that now requires an evaluation, the development of a comparison population may be impossible. Another difficulty many researchers face is that, having not been consulted in the formulation of a program, they may have to evaluate that program without a clear definition of its original objectives (for example, in evaluating the Professional Standards Review Organization program, a basic question arose as to whether its objective was to reduce Medicare expenditures or to decrease overall spending for hospital care).

Each of these three areas of health services research can be important to the policy process, in terms of (1) influencing overall policy direction, (2) helping to formulate new programs, and (3) determining the future of existing efforts. However, this potential has not been fully realized, and even where there has been a linkage between research and policy, the outcome has not always been positive. The reasons for this are complex and are as much a product of the inherent limitations of research itself as they are the fault of both researchers and policy makers. A number of points are relevant to understanding and improving the current situation.

GREAT EXPECTATIONS

First, we must realize that sometimes our expectations of what research can accomplish cannot be met. Research is, at best, an imperfect tool. It seldom proves anything; rather, it simply suggests that some hypothesis is or is not true.

The proverbial smoking gun is very seldom to be found in research. An example of this is the fact that, for 30 years, people have done research on the deleterious health effects of smoking. While most would now agree that a relationship does exist, it has taken a long time for the effects of that research to be translated into changes in public policy. Only after some clinical studies confirmed what the epidemiological research had long suggested did any changes occur. Before that, we simply had established a statistical correlation between smoking and disease.

Even now the "proof" does not stop tobacco subsidies or raise cigarette taxes to help pay for the health care costs of smokers. If there is still a debate even with all the evidence linking smoking and health, it is no wonder that we must set our expectations fairly low when dealing with other, more tenuous research findings.

One can only imagine how the policy maker's eyes glaze over when, after expecting an absolute answer from the researcher, he receives a series of qualifications and disclaimers. This is not to say that research is not useful, but to point out that what it can realistically accomplish must be understood by both the researcher and the policy maker. It will simply never be the sole basis for making decisions.

Some Consequences for the Researcher

It should be noted that, since research does not provide definitive answers, it may be used by researchers on either side of an issue to prove their respective points. For example, using the same data, two researchers may reach very different conclusions, depending upon their methodology, or what they choose to stress in those data, or their ideological bias. While one researcher might look at an increase in the poverty rate as proof of the failure of the poverty programs, another might see it as a function of other socioeconomic factors and as an argument for expanding such programs.

A corollary concern is that a lack of a statistical finding may be used by a policy maker as an argument for eliminating a program, even though this result might have been attributable to a problem with the research rather than with the actual program. Because of this, even if the researcher proves the null hypothesis (that is, statistical insignificance), he must be cautious in interpreting the policy significance of the findings. Of course, the null hypothesis may actually reflect the ineffectiveness of a program. However, it may equally reflect a problem in the methodology, or missing data, or the choice of an inaccurate or insensitive measure by a specific researcher. It may also be a function of the limited capacity of research, in general, to measure the benefits of a particular program. Thus, researchers, in their rush to publish results must (1) protect against the potential misuse of those findings, (2) be assured that their interpretations of the results are well justified, and (3) understand the inherent limitations of research.

Faculty members who teach public policy to nurses can include an awareness of these problems into their teaching by cautioning students not to accept without question the findings of any policy-related study. More important the students should learn how to pose questions and to examine from many angles the findings presented.

Some Consequences for the Policy Maker

By the same token, policy makers and advocates must also use research responsibly. They should not, for example, use research only when it suits their purposes. Too often, policy makers look for research that will support a specific point of view. It is a matter of applying the Procrustean technique: you take the facts and cut and stretch them to fit your notions. For example, the WIC program has undergone several evaluations. Supporters argue for its expansion on the basis of positive aspects of certain studies, while its detractors emphasize the less favorable results. Here research is being manipulated by the policy process, rather than contributing to it.

The fact that some policy makers are interested only in research that supports their positions can be seductive to the researcher who wants to influence public policy. Indeed, the researcher can fall into such a trap without even realizing it. Since much research is not exact science, the possibility of finding results that are "client oriented" is a real danger.

Policy makers should also be cautioned against selectively deciding whether research is or is not needed. Recently, for example, Congress passed legislation to reimburse hospitals under Medicare through the use of DRGs. That system will affect over $60 billion in expenditures this year. Congress enacted this program in the absence of any completed research on what its effect would be on hospitals, on beneficiaries, or on the quality of care. While a demonstration of DRGs was already underway in New Jersey, the federal legislation became law before that program was evaluated. In this case, public policy involving a major national program was made without any research basis in terms of whether it would be effective or whether it might help or hurt the recipient of care. It is important for faculty members to point out such situations to students, especially insofar as they demonstrate potential areas of incongruence between research and policy.

EMPHASIS ON COSTS

Research is often inappropriately used only for the purpose of determining a program's cost-effectiveness. In some cases, a program is clearly not going to save money but nevertheless may be beneficial. Thus costs should not be the sole indicator of the success or failure of a program. Very often, because we place such emphasis on costs —and because it is so hard to prove cost-effectiveness—we deem a program unsuccessful despite what research into other measures of success might have indicated.

For years, groups have been arguing in Congress that preventive services save money in the long run. However, Congress, which is dubious about spending more on prevention, wants research to prove that there will be savings. And research simply cannot prove it. Thus, an appropriate prevention program may not be funded because of an inappropriate emphasis on measuring cost-effectiveness.

For example, if anybody studied whether prevention programs for the elderly were cost-effective, they would find that these programs may, in fact, be more costly than traditional programs. The individual who stopped smoking or changed his or her life-style or nutritional habits at 55 and, as a result, did not die of a heart attack at the age of 65, may now live to 85. That person, at 85, who may be in need of expensive chronic care or who may die after a protracted and costly illness, might be more expensive to treat than he would have been had he died at 65. That does not mean that prevention is bad. Prevention is quite clearly needed, but we may not be able to prove that on the basis of cost. Does this mean we should eliminate such preventive programs?

BROADENING THE FOCUS OF RESEARCH

Research is often too narrowly focused. Much research attempts simply to establish statistical relationships (or the lack thereof) between some intervention and a specified outcome, in some instances merely because it is the only quantifiable relationship available. Thus the researcher may prove a hypothesis but ignore other factors that might place those findings in a different perspective or even alter the interpretation of those results.

For example, there is considerable debate right now over the effectiveness of prenatal care. Some recent studies have indicated that early prenatal care may not be as effective as its advocates argue or conventional wisdom has led us to believe. While the methodological approach of these studies is unquestionable, they may be providing only a partial picture. Prenatal care is a complex issue. For instance, the frequency or content of the care as it affects different population groups may be as important a consideration as whether care was available in the first trimester. Thus it is important that specific research efforts consider the range of factors that may affect outcomes and not look for convenient statistical relationships.

Research inherently focuses on the quantifiable. The researcher, however, should not ignore nonquantifiable but potentially overriding concerns. If, for example, prenatal care would be personally important to the researcher for his or her own family (and we doubt that many researchers would deny themselves or their wives such care), why make it an issue in terms of proving its effectiveness for other people? Why test it against some measures other than what we would apply to ourselves?

BRIDGING THE GAP

In citing the dangers implicit in research, we are not arguing against the need for it. Rather, we are arguing that research is a single element among a larger set of tools necessary to formulate policy. Recognizing this will benefit both the researcher and the policy maker and students of both public policy and research. Yet, as mentioned earlier, a gap continues to exist between public policy formulation and research. The reasons for this gap are important for nursing faculty teaching public policy to understand and therefore merit further discussion.

Communications Gap

One major factor contributing to this gap is a lack of communications. Policy makers, for example, do not always ask the right questions. In fact, they often do not know what questions to ask. For example, the concern over whether hospitals that treat a disproportionate share of the poor should get special treatment under the prospective payment system was incorrectly framed as a question of whether public hospitals were being inadequately reimbursed. Since not all public hospitals treat a disproportionate share of the poor, nor do all poor go to public hospitals, the researchers were addressing a spurious issue. The results were not only useless from a public policy sense; they also did a disservice to those public hospitals that do serve large numbers of poor patients.

Equally, researchers may not ask the necessary questions about what areas of research or aspects of their current work would be most helpful to the public policy process. Instead, some do research that is either of little interest to the policy process or not timely.

Additionally, researchers often speak a language that is foreign to the policy maker. Discussion of an "R-squared" or a "significant coefficient" is of little meaning or import to policy makers. There is a need for an interpreter in this process who can not only place research findings in context but also explain the policy implications of those findings. In trying to convey the results of nursing research to policy makers, nurses should strive to use simple, clear language devoid of such jargon. In addition, even such terms as "nursing diagnosis" or "nurse practitioner" may be meaningless to a non-nurse. Faculty members should help students couch their ideas in clear, comprehensible language.

Conflicting Incentives

Part of the communications problem is a function of the fact that policy makers and researchers have conflicting incentives. The policy maker requires brief, nontechnical, definitive answers. He has neither the time nor interest for more. The researcher, however, may be more concerned with preparing technical papers that will be admired by his peers and published in scientific journals. The pressures of gaining tenure and professional respect may outweigh the concerns over whether a report is useful from a policy perspective.

Poor Timing

An issue related to communications is that of timing. Researchers must anticipate what issues will be of importance to the policy process and keep their research relevant. Even when this has been done, however, the time it takes to complete the research may render the results, no matter how definitive, useless to the policy maker. Researchers must be familiar enough with the policy debate to anticipate issues and must look to the future to anticipate timely issues based on policy trends. In this way they can have sufficient lead time to carry out research.

In turn, the policy maker must wait for the research that is being done and not act precipitously. For example, although HCFA was conducting a major demonstration of the hospice program, Congress passed legislation prior to the completion of that effort. If we are to assume that the demonstration was important, the timing of the legislation appears to be inappropriate. Although we understand the political exigencies of the policy-making process, it is clear that there must be some orderly relationship between that process and research if we are to obtain the most out of research.

Dissemination

Another related problem is poor dissemination of research results. A considerable body of important research exists but is presented in journals the policy maker neither reads nor has even heard of. Only to the extent that an article is newsworthy and appears in the popular media does it ever come to the attention of the policy maker. Currently, the mechanisms that might bridge this gap (both to provide information on what research is currently being conducted and to prepare understandable, policy-relevant descriptions of results) do not exist. While groups like the Health Staff Seminar and the Association for Health Services Research do provide some linkages, there are no regular vehicles for conveying such information.

IMPLICATIONS FOR NURSING

There are important roles for nursing in integrating policy and research with other disciplines, though to date, nurses have not capitalized on their backgrounds. Policy is approved advocacy for certain needs and rights of the population. Historically, nurses have served as advocates for patients and families. Further, for decades nurses have incorporated the knowledge that socioeconomic and environmental factors have a major impact on health status and outcomes. Care has been based on a patient needs assessment in which home and community environments and economic, social, and emotional as well as medically related factors have been examined. To meet patients' needs, a multidisciplinary approach to care extending from institutional health care settings to patients' homes and communities has been employed. As such, nurses are in a unique position both to objectively interpret existing health-related research that could be useful in the development of health policy and to be involved in multi-disciplinary, policy-relevant research.

However, until recently nurses have paid little attention to health policy and also have not had sound training in research. The focus of academic nursing has been on the development of the field of nursing rather than on how nursing relates to the larger health care system. Much emphasis has been given to the development and testing of nursing theory. Even where nursing research exists, in general, the issues studied have been related to patient care and differences in patients' responses to care, factors associated with student nurse education, factors associated with nurse educators, and differences in the performance of nurses having various types of educational preparation, among others. Many times, the research designs have been weak, the sample sizes small, the results confined to nursing journals not often read by individuals in other disciplines, or presented in jargon understood only by nurses; further, the questions posed often are seen as inconsequential by policy makers. This is not to say that all research in nursing has been conducted poorly or has been misdirected. A wide variety of nursing studies certainly have been relevant to both the discipline of nursing and to wider policy issues, such as the Teaching Nursing Homes project and cost-effectiveness studies of nurses as alternative providers of care, to give but a few examples. However, studies such as those looking at the therapeutic use of touch, locus of control, and stresses faced by nurses in various settings are less likely to pique the interest of policy makers than studies examining interventions aimed at improving patients' functional status or reducing costs of care.

In terms of health policy, with the rapid changes in the health care system and the primary concerns of cost containment and the changing role of providers, nurses in conjunction with other professionals are in a strategic position to evaluate some of the impacts of these changes. Examples of such research might include the effects of early hospital discharge on the patient, family, and community in terms of health outcomes and costs; how early discharge has affected manpower needs for nurses in various health care settings; and what new types of arrangements might be required to meet the health care needs of these patients and families (e.g., day care and respite care). Also, much more outcome research is needed in the care of the elderly and low-birthweight infants, two groups consuming a large proportion of health care dollars.

CONCLUSION

The policy process can benefit immeasurably from health services research, and health services research clearly stands to benefit from having an audience of the policy makers. But both need a better means of communicating. Scientific jargon must be translated into understandable and policy-relevant information. The priorities and expectations of both the policy maker and the researcher must be conveyed. In addition, the policy maker needs a better understanding of the limitations of research, while the researcher must become cognizant of the potential for abuse of that research by advocates of particular points of view.

Such groups as the National Center for Health Services Research and the Association for Health Services Research can and do play a significant role in this process. Through conferences, publications, and newsletters, they have brought the two worlds closer together. But that is not enough. These organizations perform an ad hoc function rather than structurally closing the gap.

A different view of the researcher and the policy maker is, in our opinion, required. We often view them as though they were of different species, the "Academicus irrelevantus," and the "Politicus superficialus." Rather, they simply function in two different environments, with little understanding of each others' worlds. The need, then, is to help both of them build their own understanding of each others' worlds. The researcher must come to understand the political process and the demands it makes. The policy maker must see the uses and limitations of research.

This idea is not without precedent. In the past, the Brookings fellows—and, currently, both the Robert Wood Johnson Foundation health policy fellows and the American Association for the Advancement of Science program—have given researchers exposure to the policy-making process. Additionally, the federal government's fellowship program has permitted federal employees to spend some time in academic settings, and vice versa. Lastly, think tanks like the Urban Institute, the Brookings Institution, and the American Enterprise Institute have permitted policy makers, after they leave the government, to spend time in research settings and to help bridge that gap. These institutions, which serve as feeders to government agencies, particularly providing senior-level policy and evaluation personnel, are places where nurses should get involved as well.

Changes in the health care system are occuring with great speed. Private pressures to contain costs, combined with the deficit problems at the national level, have led to major policy chages at the federal, state, and local levels. That process will continue, and with it the increased need for research and program evaluation. The federal government and foundations must ensure that funding priorities for research reflect those changes. Efforts that help merge the experiences and priorities of the academic and political worlds must be encouraged and expanded. The nursing profession must play a more significant role in that process, and it is up to nursing faculty to take the lead.

7

RESOURCES FOR TEACHING PUBLIC POLICY

Diane O. McGivern

Nurses' participation in policy formulation, which will result in a more client-centered health care delivery system, requires preparation not previously included in baccalaureate and master's curricula. On the premise that individuals who understand the industry in which they work can exert influence, courses or lectures on health care financing, law, private- and public-sector initiatives, and politics and legislation are being offered collaboratively with other departments or taught by nursing faculty with the assistance of outside experts. Clearly, the need to provide a context for these pieces of content prompts nurse educators and practitioners to learn and then teach the process and content of health and public policy.

What are the expected outcomes for beginning and advanced students and, perhaps, for faculty? Teaching public policy is important at all levels and should not be limited to graduate programs: our goal as faculty is to develop a critical mass of nurses at all levels with the requisite knowledge and skills. Thus limiting our focus to a small percantage of nurses is self-defeating. In addition, professionals who are capable of participating in public policy may have varied levels of skills corresponding to the levels of the public policy process. The remainder of this chapter discusses these skills and the resources available to teach them to students at all levels.

THE POLICY PROCESS AND LEARNING OUTCOMES

The three levels of activities or outcomes that students can achieve parallel, to some extent, the public policy process. Policy, as a set of beliefs or general philosophy that guides and directs actions or decisions, implies a series of steps. The public policy process starts with wants and needs, perhaps not well-defined, moves to some more widely recognized and precisely defined need, which is then formulated as an issue or issues to be addressed and resolved. The policy that has been adopted and implemented will then be evaluated by some means, formally or informally.

The expected outcomes for students of public policy should correspondingly range from becoming well informed, to becoming an active participant in issue formulation, and, finally, to playing a leading role in policy implementation.

Becoming Well Informed

Since by definition public policy is the philosophically dictated course of action taken by government, it follows that, to be well informed, the student of public policy must know the elements of civics. The most common mistake in policy courses is teaching the details of issues, legislative proposals, or policy analysis to students who lack rudimentary knowledge of government. It is like teaching the difference between right- and left-sided cardiac failure to someone who has forgotten high school biology.

Becoming well informed requires the habit of reading newspapers, journals, and other materials that provide informed and expert information and thoughtful analysis. The corollary to becoming well informed is engaging in discussions of issues and exchanging opinions and facts.

The seemingly pedestrian nature of this skill is disappointing to some, but it should be a relief to those who are deterred from participating in policy or the political process because of reluctance to hold office, help draft legislation, or provide expert opinion. Lack of information generally prevents professionals from exchanging ideas with better-informed peers or providing colleagues with information or expert opinion. The practice of discussing larger issues and solutions rather than personal or institutional ones needs to be established and should follow the efforts to become well informed. Being well informed is clearly basic to the two succeeding outcomes.

Participation in Issue Formulation

Issue formulation is the process of defining and refining a problem. An issue is defined by many individuals and organizations and gains recognition by virtue of its importance to significant individuals and groups. Participation at this level can include working by oneself or in conjunction with an organization to provide information that is both substantive and experientially based, as well as participating in legislative and public information committees. Public speaking to nursing and, very importantly, non-nursing groups lends the individual's informed perspective to the articulation of the issue and proposed solutions. Speaking directly with representatives of legislators, professional and consumer organizations, foundations, candidates for office, and the media helps to define and confirm the issues and possible solutions and move issues ahead on everyone's agenda.

Implementing and Evaluating Policy

After issues are formulated and defined, the next steps are implementation and evaluation of policy. The implementation of policy is subject to the vagaries of legislative, regulatory, and fiscal oversight as well as changes in public opinion and judicial interpretation, but there is still abundant opportunity for nurses to intervene in the process. Furthermore, analysis of policy outcomes is done by means of program evaluation, which requires knowledge of statistics and quantitative analysis. Nurses who have acquired this knowledge, who ideally include most master's and doctorally prepared nurses, can make important contributions to program evaluation.

TEACHING PUBLIC POLICY

Information has more value if the person who conveys it is obviously convinced of its worth and speaks from experience. Since public policy involves both content and process, the resources necessary to teach it will be both intellectual and action-based (experiential). Course offerings should not be attempted unless the faculty has access to resources of sufficient depth and breadth to support a well-constructed policy course or content sequence. For example, library journal holdings that are limited to professional or clinical journals and local or regional newspapers are not sufficient resources for public policy discussion and study. Similarly, faculty members with little or no direct experience cannot provide the framework of participation the course requires, excellent guest speakers notwithstanding. The element that ties much of this together and makes the policy course meaningful is the instructor's ability to act as a role model for the intellectual and professional responsibility for public policy participation.

RESOURCES FOR TEACHING PUBLIC POLICY

Consistent with these three dimensions of public policy and desired student outcomes, the resources necessary to teach and learn are both content- and experience-related. Resource categories include written materials, direct experiences, and interaction with policy makers. Written information in the form of journals, books, and other documents provide a surplus of factual and analytic data.

Direct experiences can range from observing a legislative session or hearing, to an internship with a legislative staff or advocacy or lobbying group, to working in the policy group of a professional or an activist organization. These efforts are both exciting and useful to students and faculty members in removing the mystique of policy and politics and enlivening the substantive content. They do not replace the knowledge gained through exposure to the classic and contemporary works on policy.

A third category of resources, also experiential, includes exposure to and interaction with policy makers themselves. These may include faculty members, guest lecturers, and other individuals whom the students seek out for discussion, and may include officers of professional organizations, foundations, and corporations, as well as government officials and legislative staff members. All of these resource categories are essential to ensure that first faculty, then students, have a genuine preparation for this aspect of professional practice.

The following discussions of resources are, necessarily, not exhaustive but rather present representative samplings of resources available in each category: Books, newspapers and newsletters, periodicals, government documents, audiovisual aids, and direct experiences. Names and addresses for all resources (except book publishers) are provided at the end of the chapter.

Books

Following are three lists of books. "Best sellers" are the ten books most often used as texts in policy courses, according to a survey of schools of nursing (see Chapter 3). "Classics" are the standard reference works in the field, based on the same survey. Every student of policy should, ideally, be familiar with these works. The "Background Reading" list contains basic references that will provide information to both student and instructor.

Best Sellers

Aiken, L. H. (Ed.) (1981). *Health Policy and Nursing Practice*. New York: McGraw-Hill.

Aiken, L., & Gortner, S. (Eds.). (1982). *Nursing in the 1980's: Crises, Opportunities, Challenges*. Philadelphia: J.B. Lippincott.

American Nurses' Association. (1980). *Nursing: A Social Policy Statement*. Kansas City: American Nurses' Association.

Feldstein, P. (1979). *Health Care Economics*. New York: John Wiley & Sons.

Fuchs, V. (1982). *Who Shall Live? Health, Economics and Social Choices*. New York: Basic Books.

Kalisch, B. J., & Kalisch, P. A. (1982). *Politics of Nursing*. Philadelphia: J.B. Lippincott.

Litman, T. J., & Robbins, L. S. (Eds.). (1984). *Health Politics and Policy*. New York: John Wiley & Sons.

Milio, N. (1981). *Promoting Health through Public Policy*. Philadelphia: F.A. Davis.

Redman, E. (1978). *The Dance of Legislation*. New York: Simon and Schuster.

Starr, P. (1982). *The Social Transformation of American Medicine*. New York: Basic Books.

Classics

Aaron, H., & Schwartz, W. (1984). *Painful Prescription: Rationing Hospital Care*. Washington, D.C.: Brookings Institution.

Ashley, J. A. (1976). *Hospitals, Paternalism, and the Role of the Nurse*. New York: Teachers College Press.

Davis, K., & Schoen, C. (1979). *Health and the War on Poverty: A Ten Year Appraisal*. Washington, D.C.: Brookings Institution.

Dahl, R. (1976). *Modern Political Analysis*. Englewood Cliffs, NJ: Prentice-Hall.

Dror, Y. (1971). *Design for Policy Sciences*. New York: Elsevier.

Ehrenreich, B., & English, D. (1973). *Witches, Midwives and Nurses: A History of Women Healers*. Westbury, NY: The Feminist Press.

Institute of Medicine. (1983). *Nursing and Nursing Education: Public Policies and Private Actions*. Washington, D.C.: National Academy Press.

Kalisch, B. J., & Kalisch, P. A. (1978). *The Advance of American Nursing*. Boston: Little, Brown.

Knowles, J. (Ed.). (1977). *Doing Better, Feeling Worse: Health in the United States*, New York: Norton.

Lasswell, R. (1958). *Politics: Who Gets What, When, How*. New York: Peter Smith.

Lindblom, C. E. (1968). *The Policymaking Process*. Englewood Cliffs, NJ: Prentice-Hall.

Nakamura, R. & Smallwood, F. (1980). *The Politics of Policy Implementation*. New York: St. Martin's.

Navarro, V. (Ed.). (1981). *Imperialism, Health and Medicine*. Farmingdale, NY: Baywood Publishing Company.

Thompson, F. (1983). *Health Policy and the Bureaucracy*. Cambridge, MA: MIT Press.

Verba, F. and Nie, N. H. (1972). *Participation in America: Political Democracy and Social Equality*. New York: Harper & Row.

Wildavsky, A. (1979). *The Politics of the Budgetary Process*. Boston: Little, Brown.

Wildavsky, A. (1979). *Speaking Truth to Power: The Art and Craft of Policy Analysis*. Boston: Little, Brown.

Background Reading

Bagwell, M., & Clements, S. (1985). *A Political Handbook for Health Professionals*. Boston: Little, Brown.

Blau, P. M. (1967). *Exchange and Power in Social Life*. New York: John Wiley & Sons.

Christenson, R. M., Engel, A. S., Jacobs, D. N., Rejai, M., & Waltzer, H. (1972). *Ideologies and Modern Politics*. New York: Dodd, Mead.

Dye, T. R. (1976). *Policy Analysis*. Birmingham: University of Alabama Press.

Enthoven, A. (1980). *Health Plan*. Reading, MA: Addison-Wesley.

Friedson, E. (1970). *Professional Dominance: The Social Structure of Medical Care*. New York: Atherton Press.

Grissum, M., & Spengler, C. (1976). *Womanpower and Health Care*. Boston: Little, Brown.

Lindblom, C. E. (1977). *Politics and Markets*. New York: Basic Books.

Lee, P. R., Estes, C. L., & Ramsay, N. B. (Eds.). (1984). *The Nation's Health*. San Francisco: Boyd & Fraser.

Marmor, T. (1973). *The Politics of Medicare*. Chicago: Aldine Publishing Company.

Marmor, T. R., & Christianson, J. B. (1982). *Health Care Policy: A Political Economy Approach*. Beverly Hills: Sage Publications.

Mason, D., & Talbott, S. (1985). *Political Action Handbook for Nurses*. Menlo Park, CA: Addison-Wesley.

Mechanic, D. (1983). *Handbook of Health, Health Care and the Health Professions*. New York: The Free Press.

Quade, E. S. (1982). *Analysis for Public Decisions*. New York: Elsevier.

Samuelson, P. (1985). *Economics*, 12th ed. New York: McGraw-Hill.

Shaw, L. E. (Ed.). (1973). *Modern Competing Ideologies*. Lexington, KY: D.C. Heath.

Somers, A. R. (1971). *Health Care in Transition: Directions for the Future*. Chicago: Hospital Research and Educational Trust.

Somers, A. R., & Somers, H. M. (1977). *Health and Health Care Policies in Perspective*. Germantown, MD: Aspen.

Newspapers and Newsletters

Newspapers that are generally considered to be accurate reporters of information and also provide some critical analysis include *The New York Times, The Washington Post*, and *The Wall Street Journal. The Washington Post* also publishes a weekly review, *The Washington Post National Weekly Edition*, which is available at special classroom rates.

Any of these could be acceptably quoted in classroom discussion and used as references in papers or projects.

Newsletters on particular aspects of health care are published by commercial publishers, special-interest groups, and professional organizations. They provide weekly or biweekly updates on various policy issues and legislative events. They do not provide extensive background on all the topics covered but usually highlight selected topics in each issue.

Newsletters that provide both current information and some in-depth issue analysis include *Washington Report on Medicine and Health* and *Washington Report on Health Legislation*. Both are published weekly by McGraw-Hill and cover legislative and health industry developments, including personnel changes. A supplement is included in *Medicine and Health* that discusses at length an issue which merits attention and will be significant over time.

The National League for Nursing sends its members policy and legislative updates, in addition to the monthly features in *Nursing & Health Care* that cover similar topics. These reports provide detailed and lengthy descriptions and evaluations of current affairs.

Capital Update is pubished bimonthly by the Washington office of the American Nurses' Association. The legislative and government coverage is broadly restricted to topics of interest to nurses and may range from updates on the Nurse Training Act to the Federal Pay Equity Act. *The Political Nurse*, published bimonthly by the ANA Department of Political Education, covers legislative and political events, including those at the state level, that are most directly pertinent to nursing.

A newsletter published biweekly and targeted to nurses is *Legislative Network for Nurses*. This publication covers legislative and other federal, state, and significant local legislatively related action.

Private Organizations and Government Sources

A great deal of information is available from government agencies and private organizations. A host of organizations produce materials that are both general and issue specific. Some organizations whose publications are useful include the American Political Science Association, National Health Council, American Hospital Association and the state hospital associations, the American Medical Association, the Children's Defense Fund, the American Psychological Association, the American Association of Retired Persons, The Urban Institute, the American Medical Peer Review Organization, and the American Public

Health Association. Many of these publish newsletters and special reports as well as issue press releases on their current activities. In addition, many specialty and trade organizations, in both nursing and other health professions, include policy updates in their publications and publish newsletters as well. Thus one would find newsletters on home health, long-term care, preferred provider organizations, and other topics.

The Government Printing Office is the source of an extraordinary number and range of reports and records. Most federal publications are available by mail and many are free or carry a nominal charge. Many state government documents are also available that may be pertinent to national, state, and local issues.

The General Accounting Office reviews and evaluates many federal programs and activities. Reviews of various federal operations may be initiated by congressional request. The General Accounting. Office publishes a free monthly listing of reports, which is available on request.

Several other governmental and quasi-governmental agencies publish policy-related reports and other documents. The Congressional Budget Office issues analyses and estimations about the federal budget. The Congressional Research Service, a unit of the Library of Congress, provides policy analysis to members of Congess and the public. The Office of Technology Assessment examines technology and its impact on society and on public policy. Similarly, the Institute of Medicine, a division of the National Institutes of Health, is assigned by Congress to study and report on issues that have a bearing on policy decisions. Among the issues the IOM has reported on are nursing research and nursing manpower. Finally, the Prospective Payment Assessment Commission, or ProPAC, reports to Congress on the prospective payment system and sponsors research projects on various aspects of the system, including nursing issues.

Information on specific legislation can be gathered from various sources. The Senate or House Document Room will mail out, on request, a copy of a bill, public law, or committee or conference report. Legislative proposals are frequently the topic or stimulus for committee hearings. The related background material and testimony is made available in the record of the hearing several months after the close of the hearings by the committee's Publications Clerk. The *Digest of Public General Bills and Resolutions*, which is published four to five times during a congressional session, lists all bills in numerical order of introduction. The *Digest* is available at a charge from the Superintendent of Documents.

Introduction of legislation, and the congressional dialogue on legislation and other topics, is recorded verbatim in the *Congressional Record*. Single copies of an issue or annual subscriptions are available for a charge from the Superintendent of Documents. The *Federal Register*, published every business day and also available by subscription from the Superintendent of Documents, publishes all regulations issued by government agencies.

Periodicals

Periodicals focusing on, or including as a regular feature, policy, politics, and legislation have increased in recent years. The journals included here fall into four general categories: general public policy, health policy, nursing targeted, and health industry related. A source of information about the many hundreds of journals available in these fields is *Ulrich's International Periodicals Directory*, available in all libraries. This groups journals by subject matter and lists the names and addresses of their publishers, as well as subscription information. Two general public policy–focused publications are the *Congressional Quarterly* and *National Journal*. These provide the most current information and analysis available on issues and policy outcomes. The *Congressional Quarterly* also publishes the *Guide to Congress*, an excellent general reference book that includes the origins, development, and current functioning of Congress. A third source of information is *The American Political Science Review*, although the content may be too narrowly focused for beginning policy students.

A number of journals focus on health policy broadly defined. For example, articles addressing the roles of state and local government in health or defining government's responsibility for public health have as much to do with government's policy process as they do with general welfare. Several journals in this category are noteworthy: *Health Affairs, Milbank Memorial Fund Quarterly, Journal of Public Health Policy, American Journal of Public Health, Journal of Health Policy, Politics and Law, Public Administration Review, Social Policy, Public Choice, Journal of Policy Analysis and Management, Policy Sciences, and Policy Studies.*

Published quarterly by Project Hope, *Health Affairs* describes itself as "a multidisciplinary journal dedicated to the serious exploration of major domestic and international health policy issues and activities of concern to society." Experts from the government, academic, and private sectors provide analyses of a wide variety of issues.

The *Health and Society* provides, four times a year, expert presentation of a chosen topic, such as altruism and organ donation, abuse and neglect in nursing homes, or costs related to asbestosis.

The American Journal of Public Health, published monthly as the official journal of the American Public Health Association, includes articles on subjects ranging from microbes to FDA regulation to WIC program participation. Regular features include public health law and public health history.

The number and focus of nursing journals have expanded in recent years, and almost all include legislative notes or articles on legislative and policy-related topics. Several of note include *Nursing Economics, Nursing & Health Care*, and *Nursing Outlook*. In addition, almost all nursing specialty journals contain updates on policy issues of interest to their readership.

Nursing Economics, published by Jannetti, Inc., contains a range of articles that deal directly or indirectly with policy issues and frequently are written by policy participants and service providers. *Nursing & Health Care*, the official publication of the National League for Nursing, has regular features and articles that focus directly on policy development and issue analysis. Regular features include "Washington Focus," which discusses issues of importance to nursing and health policy. Articles cover a range of subjects, such as education, history, and curriculum. Usually at least one or two articles per bimonthly issue cover policy and legislation information.

Nursing Outlook, a bimonthly publication of the American Journal of Nursing Company, reports on professional activities and topics of general interest to educators and practitioners, many of which have policy implications.

Industry-related publications also offer description and analyses of a range of issues affecting the health care industries. Examples of such publications include *Modern Healthcare* and *Inquiry*. *Modern Healthcare*, published biweekly, focuses on the external and institutional developments affecting hospitals and nursing homes. Features cover legislation, insurance, technology, law, and economics.

Inquiry, published four times a year by the Blue Cross and Blue Shield Association, includes papers on current health care financing concerns. Other journals on health economics include *Health Care Financing Review*, a quarterly published by HCFA; the *Journal of Economic Issues*; and *Economics and Business*.

Audiovisual Materials

Audiovisual materials to augment other types of presentations can easily be developed by faculty from the resources already discussed.

Some films and videocassette presentations have been prepared by organizations and institutions; however, unless they are very general the information may become outdated quickly, which may make them expensive short-term investments.

A limited variety of useful materials is available, however. These include NLN's videotape, *DRGs: A New Era for Nursing*; the ANA's videotape, *Nurses, Politics, and Public Policy*, available from state nurses' associations; as well as the slide package on basic policy and political concepts that accompanies this publication. Other organizations, such as women's political organizations (the League of Women Voters and the National Women's Education Fund) and trade and professional organizations publish audiovisual materials on the how-tos of politics.

Direct Experiences

Interested students at the undergraduate and graduate levels can participate in a policy, legislative, or political experience to confirm an interest or obtain experiential learning. Such experiences can range from a relatively short-term observation to a lengthy, formal internship or fellowship.

All students should be encouraged to take advantage of these opportunities, since the tasks inherent in the policy process can accommodate many skills. Students can be productively involved by preparing bibliographies, gathering supportive documentation, meeting with constituent groups, developing responses to issue inquiries, or working to advance various issues or develop policy proposals. Some suggested activities are included in the model course in Chapter 3 and in the *Student Workbook* that accompanies this book.

Individually Arranged Experiences. With faculty assistance, students can arrange short-term experiences tailored to their interests and abilities. Many legislators' offices and professional or advocacy organizations will accept individual students for volunteer work at such tasks as retrieving and arranging information. Short-term, individually arranged student experiences provide a relatively narrow view of the policy process, but most policy participants have fairly narrow fields of pursuit, such as child health, specific legislation such as Medicare and Medicaid, or professional or occupational concerns such as nursing education or practice regulation.

Contact with the Congressional Placement Office for an internship with a member of Congress and application through that office may result in a summer experience. However, other avenues of contact are available. Academic institutions have begun to develop their own federal or state liaison offices, which may help students to gain access to congressional office or committee contacts. Eventually the faculty liaison will have working knowledge of likely possibilities to match with students' requests. Organizations that offer informal placements include the American Nurses' Association Washington office, the National Hospice Organization, the National Governors Association, and the National Advisory Council on Women's Educational Programs.

Formal Offerings. Organizations and legislative offices increasingly are defining specific criteria and times for competitive applications for a publicized experience. Many specialty nursing organizations that have Washington offices offer internships in public policy for nurses. Stimulating interest and advising students on the preparation of applications or credentials are important faculty roles.

The American Association of Colleges of Nursing offers a limited number of internships through its Office of Governmental Relations, and although there is a formal application process, the actual experience is individually arranged for a minimum of four weeks. Preference is given to graduate students.

Graduate students with an interest in aging should apply to the American Association of Retired Persons' Washington office. Internships are supported with a small stipend and last up to six months. Students whose undergrduate program included strong background in policy writing or liberal arts may apply to the American Hospital Association or directly to the American Society for Nursing Service Administrators.

Opportunities for Doctorally Prepared Professionals. Formal and informal opportunities for practitioners with advanced preparation parallel the students'. Constraints for faculty are not too different from those of students, namely, providing for the time and resources such an opportunity requires. Institutional commitment to teaching public policy should be reflected in assistance provided to selected faculty who will participate on a more informed level as a result. Organizations which offer experiences for professionals with advanced academic preparation and some experience include government agencies, associations, and foundations.

The American Association of Political Science offers a relatively large number of fellowships every year to a broad spectrum of professionals.

The American Association for the Advancement of Science offers the AAAS Congressional Science and Engineering Fellows Program. Each year approximately 60 fellows, sponsored by various scientific societies, function as members of congressional staff after an initial orientation.

A similar format is followed by the Robert Wood Johnson Health Policy Fellowship program, which is designed for midcareer academics. Fellows bring back to their institutions and professional activities the policy knowledge and experience gained through the fellowship. This very competitive program offers an annual stipend and is directed through the Institute of Medicine.

White House Fellowships are one-year paid competitive internships. Several nurses have been selected in the last few years.

Policy Makers and Participants

Equally important with content and direct participation is the opportunity to meet and talk with individuals who work in policy development and implementation at the local, regional, or national level. Such individuals may represent government, private industry, the not-for-profit sector, advocacy groups, or health-related organizations.

Their representation of their agency or institution, their own role in policy development, and their knowledge of the history and development of various issues and policies provide an important element in students' understanding of one policy or a range of policies. From discussions with policy makers, students gain an understanding of the complexity and unpredictability of policy development and an appreciation for the contributions of significant participants. Students gain new perspectives and realistic understanding of political, legislative, and policy activity.

A public policy course is described elsewhere in this book (Chapter 3). It is important to use these experts within the context of a fully defined course in a lecture/discussion format. Public policy is effected on all levels of government, although emphasis tends to be placed on the federal government. It is essential to broaden the scope to include local and state policy formulation, particularly in an era in which devolution of responsibilities to the state level is emphasized.

It is always a pleasant surprise to discover the extent to which elected and appointed policy makers are willing to share their experiences and policy agendas. Any official or staff member whose role, identified interest, committee assignment, or legislative or electoral agenda makes the individual an expert on relevant issue is a potential candidate for an invitation.

Your ability to secure the speakers you desire is determined by your own participation in issues or policy discussion, the relevance of your institutional or organizational affiliation to the constituency of the policy maker, and timing (the legislative calendar and policy agenda). A joint invitation with another group may make the engagement more attractive to the speaker. Other considerations include scheduling and preparation necessary.

Generally, political and legislative calendars are extremely full and subject to much change. Conflicts frequently occur and precedence goes to the speaker's primary legislative or political concerns. Scheduling early in the morning, late in the evening, or on a weekend increases the chance that your group can be accommodated. It is also a good idea to schedule your meeting in conjunction with the policy maker's other local commitments or take your students to the policy maker.

No policy maker should be expected to offer basic instruction to you or your students; their role is to provide expert opinion. Therefore, students should already be familiar with the background of the issue and the invited speaker's role in the issue and policy debate. The experience will be far more productive if the students' preparation allows for a lively discussion between speaker and group.

The students' interaction with the policy maker has several important effects. First, issues and solutions take on an air of vital, much more immediate importance when they are enlivened by a participant's personal descriptions. Second, by discovering the extent to which policy formulation is a product of political, social, economic, and serendipitous events, students appreciate that not everything is predetermined. Third, students learn that, as citizens and well-educated professionals, their questions and appraisals are as important as anyone else's in policy formulation. These are all valuable lessons.

CONCLUSION

Many resources can be used to teach the content and process of policy formulation. Written materials provide description and analysis of issues and policy implementation and evaluation. Students can learn about public policy formulation through written resources, but learning is enhanced by direct experiences and interaction with policy participants and analyzers. One resource category does not substitute for another; all of these resources combine to support a strong public policy offering.

RESOURCE LIST

The following listings include all the resources mentioned in this chapter, except for books and book publishers. The following references provide additional general information:

Bradham, D. D. (1985, May–June). Health policy formulation and analysis. *Nursing Economics, 3,* 167–72.

Collins, J. B., Richie, S., & Vines, D. W. (1983). Nursing and policy making: Washington fellowships. *Nursing Economics, 1,* 54–58.

Vase, C. (1975). *A guide to library sources in political science: American government.* Washington, DC: American Political Science Association.

Newspapers

The New York Times
229 West 43rd Street
New York, NY 10036

The Washington Post
Mail Subscription Department
1150 15th Street, N.W.
Washington, D.C. 20071
(800) 424-9203

The Wall Street Journal
200 Burnett Road
Chicopee, MA 01021
(413) 592-7761

Washington Post National Weekly Edition
1150 15th Street, N.W.
Washington, D.C. 20071
(800) 624-2367 ext. 4280

Newsletters

Washington Report on Medicine & Health
and
Washington Report on Health Legislation
McGraw-Hill Book Company
1120 Vermont Avenue, N.W.
Suite 1200
Washington, D.C. 20005

Legislative Updates and other periodic publications
National League for Nursing
10 Columbus Circle
New York, NY 10019-1350

Capital Update
ANA Washington Office
1101 14th Street, N.W.
Washington, D.C. 20005

The Political Nurse
ANA Department of Political Education
1101 14th Street, N.W.
Washington, D.C. 20005

Legislative Network for Nurses
Legislative Network for Nursing, Inc.
P.O. Box 44071
L'Enfant Plaza, S.W.
Washington, D.C. 20026

Private Organizations and Government Sources

American Association of Retired Persons
1909 K Street, N.W.
Washington, D.C. 20049
(202) 872-4700

American Hospital Association
444 North Capitol Street, N.W.
Suite 500
Washington, D.C. 20001
(202) 638-1100

American Medical Association
1101 Vermont Avenue, N.W.
Washington, D.C. 20005
(202) 789-7400

American Medical Peer Review Association
440 First Street, N.W.
Suite 500
Washington, D.C. 20001
(202) 628-1853

American Political Science Association
  1527 New Hampshire Avenue, N.W.
  Washington, D.C. 20036
  (202) 483-2512

American Psychological Association
  1200 17th Street, N.W.
  Washington, D.C. 20036
  (202) 955-7660

American Public Health Association
  1015 15th Street, N.W.
  Washington, D.C. 20005
  (202) 789-5600

Children's Defense Fund
  122 C Street, N.W.
  Suite 400
  Washington, D.C. 20001
  (202) 628-8787

Congressional Budget Office
  HOB Annex #2
  Washington, D.C. 20515
  (202) 226-2600

Congressional Record, Federal Register, Digest of Public General Bills and Resolutions
  Superintendent of Documents
  Government Printing Office
  Washington, D.C. 20402
  (202) 783-3238

Congressional Research Service
  101 Independence Avenue, S.E.
  Washington, D.C. 20540
  (202) 287-5700

General Accounting Office
  Headquarters:
  441 G Street, N.W.
  Washington, D.C. 20548
  (202) 275-2812 (Office of Public Information/Press)
  Ordering reports:
  P.O. Box 6015

Gaithersburg, MD 20877
(202) 275-6241

Government Printing Office
Superintendent of Documents
710 North Capitol Street, N.W.
Washington, D.C. 20402
(202) 275-3204 (information)
(202) 783-3238 (publications orders and inquiries)

House Document Room
H226, Capitol
Washington, D.C. 20515
(202) 225-3456

Institute of Medicine
2101 Constitution Avenue, N.W.
Washington, D.C. 20418
(202) 334-2169

National Health Council, Inc.
622 Third Avenue
New York, NY 10017
(212) 972-2700

Office of Technology Assessment
U.S. Congress
Washington, D.C. 20540
(202) 287-5580

Prospective Payment Assessment Commission
300 Seventh Street, S.W.
Washington, D.C. 20024
(202) 453-3986

Senate Document Room
SH-BO4
Senate Hart Office Building
Washington, D.C. 20510
(202) 224-7860

The Urban Institute
2100 M Street, N.W.
Washington, D.C. 20037
(202) 833-7200

Periodicals

American Journal of Public Health
American Public Health Association
1015 15th Street, N.W.
Washington, D.C. 20005
(202) 789-5600

The American Political Science Review
American Political Science Association
1527 New Hampshire Avenue, N.W.
Washington, D.C. 20036
(202) 483-2512

Congressional Quarterly Service and *Guide to Congress*
Weekly Report
Congressional Quarterly, Inc.
1414 22nd Street, N.W.
Washington, D.C. 20037

Economics and Business Letter
Slippery Rock State College
Department of Economics and Business
Slippery Rock, PA 16057

Health Care Financing Review
Health Care Financing Administration
Department of Health & Human Services
East High Rise Building, Room 365
6401 Security Blvd.
Baltimore, MD 21207
(310) 597-3000
Subscriptions to:
Superintendent of Documents
Washington, D.C. 20402

Health Affairs
Project HOPE
Millwood, VA 22646
(703) 837-2100

Inquiry
Blue Cross & Blue Shield Association
676 North St. Clair Street
Chicago, IL 60611

Subscriptions to:
Box 527
Glenview, IL 60025

J.E.I. (Journal of Economic Issues)
Association for Evolutionary Economics
c/o F. Gregory Hayden
Department of Economics
University of Nebraska
Lincoln, Nebraska 68588
(202) 822-7845

Journal of Health Politics, Policy and Law
Duke University
Department of Health Administration
Box 3018
Durham, NC 27710
(919) 684-4188

Journal of Policy Analysis and Management
Association for Public Policy Analysis and Management
John Wiley & Sons, Inc.
605 Third Avenue
New York, NY 10016
(202) 692-6000

Journal of Public Health Policy
Journal of Public Health Policy, Inc.
23 Pheasant Way
South Burlington, VT 05401

Millbank Memorial Fund Quarterly
Cambridge University Press
510 North Avenue
New Rochelle, NY 10801
(914) 235-0300

Modern Healthcare
Crain Communications
740 Rush Street
Chicago, IL 60611

National Journal
  Government Research Corporation
  1730 M Street, N.W.
  Washington, D.C. 20036
  (202) 857-1400

Nursing Economics
  Anthony J. Jannetti, Inc.
  North Woodbury Road
  Box 56
  Pitman, NJ 08071
  (609) 589-2319

Nursing & Health Care
  National League for Nursing
  10 Columbus Circle
  New York, NY 10019-1350
  (212) 582-1022

Nursing Outlook
  American Journal of Nursing Company
  555 West 57th Street
  New York, NY 10019
  (212) 582-8820

Policy Sciences
  Elsevier Scientific Publications Company
  Box 211
  1000 AE Amsterdam
  Netherlands

Policy Studies Review
  Policy Studies Organization
  University of Illinois
  361 Lincoln Hall
  Urbana, IL 61801
  (217) 359-8541

Public Administration Review
  American Society for Public Administration
  1120 G Street, N.W.
  Suite 500
  Washington, D.C. 20005
  (202) 393-7878

Public Choice
Kluwer Academic Publishers Group
Distribution Center
Box 322
3300 AH Dordrecht
Netherlands

Social Policy
Social Policy Corporation
33 West 42nd Street
New York, NY 10036
(212) 840-7619

Audiovisual Materials

DRGs: A New Era for Nursing (videotape)
National League for Nursing
10 Columbus Circle
New York, NY 10019-1350

Nurses, Politics, and Public Policy (videotape)
American Nurses' Association
2420 Pershing Road
Kansas City, MO 64108
(816) 474-5720
(also available from the state nurses' association)

League of Women Voters of the United States
1730 M Street, N.W.
Washington, D.C. 20036
(202) 429-1965

National Women's Educational Fund
1410 Q Street, N.W.
Washington, D.C. 20009
(202) 462-8606

Experiences

American Association for the Advancement of Science
AAAS Congressional Science & Engineering Fellows Program
1515 Massachusetts Avenue, N.W.
Washington, D.C. 20005
(202) 467-4400

American Association of Colleges of Nursing
One Dupont Circle
Suite 530
Washington, D.C. 20036
(202) 463-6930

American Association of Retired Persons
1909 K Street, N.W.
Washington, D.C. 20049
(202) 872-4700

American Hospital Association
444 North Capitol Street, N.W.
Suite 550
Washington, D. C. 20001
(202) 638-1100

American Nurses' Association
Washington Office
1101 14th Street, N.W.
Suite 200
Washington, D.C. 20005
(202) 789-1800

American Political Science Association
1527 New Hampshire Avenue, N.W.
Washington, D.C. 20036
(202) 483-2512

American Society for Nursing Service Administration
840 North Lakeshore Drive
Chicago, IL 60611
(312) 280-6410

National Advisory Council on Women's Educational Programs
425 13th Street, N.W.
Washington, D.C. 20004
(202) 376-1038

National Governors Association
444 North Capitol Street
Suite 250
Washington, D.C. 20001
(202) 624-5300

National Hospice Organization
    1901 North Fort Meyer Drive
    Suite 402
    Arlington, VA 22209
    (202) 243-5900

Robert Wood Johnson Policy Fellowship Program
    Institute of Medicine
    2101 Constitution Avenue
    Washington, D.C. 20418
    (202) 389-6891

White House Fellowship Program
    712 Jackson Place, N.W.
    Washington, D.C. 20503
    (202) 395-4522

8

LINKING PRACTICE WITH PUBLIC POLICY: USING THE CASE STUDY METHOD TO TEACH PUBLIC POLICY

Susan C. Roe

If nurses are to attain a leadership role in the public policy arena, a solid knowledge base in all aspects of health care policy is essential. Knowledge and understanding, however, are not enough. Of equal importance is mastery of skills in policy analysis.

Policy analysis requires the development of analytic thinking, conceptualization skills, and a repertoire of problem-solving approaches (Lynn, 1980). Active involvement in the policy process gives nurses the opportunity to achieve these necessary competencies. Therefore, the education of nurses who seek to participate in public policy should encompass a variety of teaching and learning strategies.

A knowledge base is often best developed through lecture and discussion coupled with a requirement for background and preparatory reading. The case study method presents real-world health care policy problems in which nursing students can, in a simulated situation, master analytic thought and build their expertise in problem solving.

This chapter offers nursing faculty members necessary guidelines for effective use of the case study method. A brief overview of the case study method is included as a framework so that nursing students are able to gain maximum benefit. Two health care policy cases studies follow. Included are case questions that will aid students in their analysis. Suggestions for integrating these case studies into a health policy course can be found in Chapter 3.

THE CASE STUDY METHOD: A FORM OF EXPERIENTIAL LEARNING

Students seem to learn best by doing. The case study method offers an opportunity for "vicarious living and learning" for students who need to know how to make decisions using logic and analytical skills (Ronstadt, 1977, p. 1). This form of experiential learning goes beyond the traditional methods, which tend to contribute only to the understanding of skills and not to their development (Hanson, 1981).

Kolb (1984) defines experiential learning as the process whereby knowledge is created through the transformation of experience (p. 38). The process is seen as a four-stage cycle that incorporates four adaptive learning modes: concrete experience, reflective observation, abstract conceptualization, and active experimentation. While Kolb's model suggests that concrete experience/abstract conceptualization and active experimentation/reflective observation are dialectically opposed adaptive orientations, however, learning lies in the interaction between these modes and the way in which the dialectics get resolved.

The learning process operates as a feedback loop. Concrete experience initiates the cycle. The nursing student thinks about, observes, and reflects upon a concrete experience by identifying the similarities, differences, patterns, and trends found in that experience. The student applies the observations and reflections by making generalizations and formulating principles and concepts. Active experimentation follows, in an attempt to determine if the principles and concepts are valid. This experimentation leads the student to another concrete experience. As a result, knowledge is gained from both grasping and transforming the concrete experience.

A recent interview study of policy makers, researchers, and staff developers that examined assumptions about adult learning (Lambert, 1984) affirms Kolb's (1984) premise about experiential learning. This study revealed that if an activity cannot be assigned meaning, learning does not occur. Meaning can be established by the interaction of experience and purpose and must be processed through self-reflection, analysis, and critique.

The case study is a written document used to stimulate this type of learning. The case study method involves the student in three interdependent stages of activity: reading and contemplating the case, analyzing and discussing the case with fellow students, and reflecting attitudes toward the case (Berquist & Phillips, 1981). In this manner, the objective of the case study method—facilitating the development of skills in assessment, analysis, and conceptualization necessary for effective problem solving—is achieved. In addition, insights into the policy process, which are often gained over a long period of time, can rather quickly become part of the student's repertoire. The case study method can therefore be a blend of didactic and experiential learning.

Obviously, the main advantage of the case study method is the development of analytical and general thought processes. These are essential for dealing with public policy issues. Specific sharpening of skills in situation assessment, problem diagnosis, evaluation of alternatives, and identification and formulation of workable plans to implement recommendations can also generalize to other nursing activities (Rakich, Longest & Darr, 1983).

One could contend that superficiality is one possible pitfall when using the case study method. Spending a few hours analyzing a case may not yield a better learning environment than studying analytical skills without the benefit of a case study (Lynn, 1980). What makes the difference between simply studying skills and skills development is the depth of analysis required and the degree to which the case study is processed in the classroom.

USING THE CASE STUDY METHOD

While case studies may be executed through role playing, debates, field experiences, and panels (Applegate & Entrekin, 1984), group involvement appears to yield the most dynamic results. The group forum, which may be either structured or unstructured, allows for the most productive skills development (Rakich, Longest & Darr, 1983).

Classroom techniques for case study presentation are determined by the faculty. Case study presentations should always identify the key points about the case. Then, primary alternatives should be discussed, along with recommendations for specific action.

An unstructured or semistructured approach to case studies gives students the opportunity to prepare the case either individually or in a group. Class discussion is initiated by the faculty member by using open-ended questions addressed to the whole class or to individual students. A lead-off question, which is general in nature, focuses on the issues involved in the case, the variables to be considered, and what alternative actions might be selected. This case study approach requires that the instructor prepare before class by predetermining the major areas of the case the students should analyze. Once in the classroom, encouraging differing lines of thought and argument will be important for helping the students understand the different possibilities of the case in question (Berquist & Phillips, 1981).

A structured approach incorporates written analyses, either done individually or in a group, that are formally presented in the classroom. A general discussion by the entire class follows. Which approach to use generally depends on faculty preference, class size and length, and the instructor's and students' familiarity with the case study method (Rakich, Longest & Darr, 1983).

Students will have more success with the case study method if they prepare adequately and if both instructor and students have effective listening skills. Preparation enables students to share what they have learned and increases their willingness to subject their ideas to open debate and criticism.

To prepare, the student should read each case study at least three times. The first reading focuses on the situation or the presenting problems as well as the key players. At this point, the student should operationally define the issues and problems involved in the case. On the second reading, the student makes notes reflecting her assessment of the issue presented. If the case study contains exhibits, the student examines them for their purpose and relevance to the case. Important considerations should be separated from unimportant ones. Reasonable assumptions should be made when information is absent. Appropriate disciplines and methodologies should be applied. The third reading takes place before the case is presented in class. Its purpose is to ensure that the student has considered all pertinent information.

Analysis of each case should be broad. Rather than merely answering the assigned questions, students should begin case analysis with a fundamental query, "What are the key issues in this case?" The main alternatives or options involved in the case should then be assessed based on the key issues and the assigned questions.

Finally, the focus of the analysis should be determined. Then each option is analyzed, and discrete recommendations are made and implementation strategies are decided on. Since cases do not have one right answer, students must be able to justify their decisions: in other words, their decisions must be seen to derive from the initial premises.

Usually, distinguishing relevant facts is preferable to analyzing every fact available. Several types of analysis can be attempted:

1. *Comprehensive analysis*, using quantitative and qualitative data

to support recommendations for action based on in-depth analysis of key issues.

2. *Specialized analysis*, used as an in-depth treatment of a single question or issue.
3. *Lead-off analysis*, focusing on discussion of an initial question asked about the case or the case's major issues.
4. *Hit-and-run analysis*, used as a generalized treatment of assigned questions or major issues.
5. *Integrating analysis*, using information from supplementary sources to enrich the analysis (Ronstadt, 1977; Rakich, Beaufort & Darr, 1983; Berquist & Phillips, 1981).

The case study method requires active involvement by both students and faculty members. The classroom is viewed as a world of ideas in which students are able to develop necessary skills in health care policy analysis by having the opportunity to make decisions as if they were in the "real world."

HEALTH CARE POLICY CASE STUDIES

The two case studies that are included in this chapter can be used in any graduate-level nursing health care policy course. Each case study includes a description of the policy issue or problem, the key players, supplementary information, and case questions. The case studies are designed to fit in classes 11 and 12 of the model course presented in Chapter 3 but may be used in a variety of contexts. Additional references may be found at the end of the chapter.

Case Study 1: Baby Doe

Mandating life-sustaining measures for severely disabled newborns

This case study covers an emergent health care policy concern: What is the appropriate role of the government in determining health care delivery practice? To what extent should the government be involved in clinical decision making? Should federal and state governments impose a definition of what is right for society even if it conflicts with an individual family's wishes? The far-reaching effect of these issues is demonstrated by the fact that attempts to resolve them have involved all three branches of government: executive, legislative, and judicial.

Background. Discussions of the merits of employing life-sustaining measures for severely disabled newborns are not new. Historically, these discussions took place privately between health care professionals and family members. In 1982, these private matters became a matter of public concern. In Bloomington, Indiana, the parents of an infant born with Down's syndrome and a detached esophagus made the decision, in consultation with health care professionals, to withhold from the baby life-sustaining surgical treatment. The reasons given were their reluctance to prolong the life of an infant that would no doubt meet an inevitable early death, as well as the extensive health care services that would be required to support the disabled child. Although these considerations seemed reasonable to the parents of "Baby Doe," as well as to other parents who have faced a similar decision, the Reagan administration took exception.

Prompted by the Baby Doe case, the Department of Health and Human Services (DHHS) issued interim regulations in March 1983 regarding health care of handicapped infants. The regulations required hospitals to post in a "conspicuous place" a notice stating that, under Section 504 of the Rehabilitation Act of 1973, it is unlawful for hospitals receiving federal assistance to withhold life-sustaining treatment from a handicapped infant. They were also required to post a telephone hotline number for reporting of suspected violations of the law.

Opposition to the regulations was registerd by numerous professional health care organizations, including the American Hospital Association, the American Medical Association, the ANA, the American Academy of Pediatrics, the American College of Obstetricians and Gynecologists, and the Nurses Association of the American Academy of Obstetricians and Gynecologists. This marked the first time in recent years that physicians, nurses, hospital administrators, and other health professionals have been so united in a common cause. They objected to the government's interference in clinical practice and argued that the rules did not give appropriate consideration to parents' wishes. They also pointed out that the regulations were issued with only a 15-day comment period, as opposed to the minimum of 30 days required by the Administrative Procedures Act.

In a legal challenge spearheaded by the American Academy of Pediatrics, the U.S. District Court judge for the District of Columbia described the interim rules as "arbitrary and capricious" and criticized DHHS Secretary Margaret Heckler for not appearing to give adequate consideration to the pros and cons of relying on the wishes of parents. The judge also objected to the abbreviated comment period.

After the initial set of rules was invalidated, DHHS published revised regulations and asked for public comment. The revisions still had not addressed the issues that were previously in question: government interference in clinical decision making and family wishes. At this time (November 1983), a baby was born in Stony Brook, New York, with spina bifida and hydrocephalus. In addition to the questions raised by the original Baby Doe case and the government's subsequent action, the so-called Baby Jane Doe case raised the question of whether withholding treatment to a handicapped newborn could be considered discriminatory and, furthermore, whether the government could have access to medical records in cases of possible discrimination. DHHS was denied access to this infant's records, since it was ruled and upheld that there had been no discrimination and therefore no violation.

Final regulations regarding the mandating of treatment for severely disabled newborns were issued by DHHS in January 1984. The rules included the posting of notices, the use of voluntary Infant Care Review Committees (ICRCs), and the establishment of a hotline to be used only after either the ICRC or the state child protective agency had been notified. As summarized by Secretary Heckler, the federal government was to be the "protector of last resort."

The issue has been carried over into the legislative arena as well. In 1984 Congress passed an amendment to the Child Abuse Prevention and Treatment Act that applied the definition of child abuse to cases where seriously handicapped infants were denied life-sustaining treatment. The Baby Doe provision included a detailed definition of "withholding of medically indicated treatment" that would instruct physicians, hospitals, and nurses as to when such treatment must be provided. The bill also required states that participate in the child abuse grant program to set up procedures or programs to respond to reports of medical neglect, including the withholding of medically indicated treatment. President Reagan signed the amendment on October 4, 1984.

DHHS published its final rules implementing the legislation on April 15, 1985. The final regulations were revised based on arguments from ANA and other groups that government should not further define "withholding of medically indicated treatment." Instead, DHHS included the definitions as interpretive guidelines without the binding force of law. The legislation gives doctors and families the right to decide when it is appropriate to withhold care, even though the government monitors their activities.

As a result of the DHHS regulations, the states are in a position to implement their own programs, and many have done so. Louisiana was the first to sign into law the mandating of treatment for handicapped newborns.

Even though the issue has progressed in the legislative and regulatory arenas, it is still pending in the Supreme Court, which has agreed to review, during the 1985–86 term, whether Section 504 is applicable to Baby Doe cases. If the Court decides that it is, there will be two applicable pieces of legislation for cases involving disabled newborns.

Government has acted, but questions still remain. Both sides feel that they have won to a certain extent: government and right-to-life groups are pleased that action has been taken; health care professionals are pleased that they have limited the extent to which government can intervene. The issue will continue to be debated, and government, practitioners, and families are sure to be confronted with it in the future.

Case Study Questions. The following questions can be selected for use as they best fit with either course or individual objectives. Analysis of the case study can be carried out in either a structured or unstructured format.

1. What are the health care policy problems raised by the Baby Doe case study? Outline the major positions taken by those who support the government's stand and by those who oppose it.
2. What specific protective responsibilities does society have to individuals and to society as a whole? What role does society play in curbing government's interference? What level of government (e.g., state or federal) should be responsible?
3. What interest groups were involved in the Baby Doe controversy? To what extent were they successful in achieving their ends? Why were certain groups more or less successful than others?
4. What are the "politics" of the Baby Doe case? Who stands to lose or gain in this situation? Were there any underlying reasons, ideological or political, for the government to step in?
5. What policy implications arise when the government becomes involved in social, moral, or ethical decision making?
6. What policy alternatives could the government have used other than regulation?
7. Given that the federal and state governments are mandating

that care be provided to severely disabled newborns, how can this policy decision best be implemented? Who should be involved?

8. What role can nurses play in the decision-making procedures mandated by the Baby Doe regulations? What information regarding health policy and law should a nurse provide to the parents of a severely disabled newborn?

9. How much influence should interest groups have? Which groups should take precedence: those with the greatest number of adherents? those with the greatest technical expertise? those whose beliefs are in line with administrative policies?

Case Study 2

Nurse-midwifes: Policy implications of the crisis in the insurance industry

This case study addresses some of the issues that can arise when a profession expands its scope of practice. This case has implications for all nurses in advanced practice but focuses on certified nurse-midwives, who for the most part have been successful in securing acceptance for their role within the health care system. However, despite their cost-effectiveness, high quality of care, and a historically low rate of liability claims, nurse-midwives have been subject to events beyond the realm of nursing practice but very much affecting their practice nonetheless.

The core of this case study is the current loss of malpractice insurance facing nurse-midwives. The situation of the nurse-midwives raises many important policy questions: To what extent should professional associations bring to the attention of government seemingly unfair practices in the private sector, especially if those practices result from forces in the economy that were not directly caused by previous government action? In other words, at what point should a problem move from the private into the public sector? As the trend continues for more nurses to practice independently, what will be the effects of the insurance crisis on other nursing specialty groups? How can they ensure that what has happened to the nurse-midwives will not happen to them, and what can they do to support the nurse-midwives?

Background. In 1955, a small group of nurse-midwives established the American College of Nurse-Midwifery (now called the American College of Nurse Midwives, or ACNM); in 1985, there were an estimated 2,500 nurse-midwives in the United States, most of whom practice under their state's nurse practice act.

The growth in numbers of nurse-midwives and the scope of their practice is impressive. It is estimated that 3 percent of the babies in the United States are delivered by nurse-midwives, 80 percent of whom have at least a baccalaureate degree. Nurse-midwives work in clinical collaboration with physicians under written alliance and protocol agreements that establish mechanisms for consultation and referral. ACNM has an agreement with the American College of Obstetricians and Gynecologists outlining guidelines for working relationships. Approximately 75 percent of the births attended by certified nurse-midwives (CNMs) take place in hospitals; another 15 percent take place in accredited birthing centers.

The place the CNMs have created for themselves within the health care system was jeopardized when, in May 1985, the ACNM was notified that its blanket malpractice insurance policy, which covered the approximately 1,400 CNMs in independent practice, would not be renewed on July 1 because of the unavailability of reinsurance. Then, in July, the insurance company further cancelled all policies that had been written after January 1, 1985. Over the next several months, ACNM contacted 17 other insurance companies but was unable to obtain insurance for its members, in spite of the nurse-midwives' low incidence of lawsuits (only 6 percent of CNMs have been sued, compared to 60 percent of obstetricians).

Indeed, this crisis for the nurse-midwives is believed to be not a result of any actions on their part but rather of a general crisis in the insurance industry that had its origin in the 1970s. During that time of high interest rates, insurance companies were eager to write policies so that they could invest the premiums at the prevailing rates of nearly 20 percent. At the same time, to attract customers, insurance premiums were kept low. In the early 1980s, this led to a crisis situation when, simultaneously, interest rates dropped sharply; insurance losses, and thus the companies' payouts, increased just as sharply; and the unrealistically low premiums failed to cover the difference. This situation is affecting several other groups, including architects, truckers, asbestos workers, towns and municipalities, and day care centers, as well as nurse-midwives, as insurance companies raise premiums and attempt to minimize risks by not writing policies

After attempting to place their insurance with other insurance companies, ACNM pursued several other paths toward resolution of the problem. First they took the case to the states, which are responsible for regulating the insurance industry: individual nurse-midwives contacted their state insurance commissioners, legislators, and other officials. Only one state, New Jersey, was able to offer insurance through a private carrier. In other states, CNMs have obtained coverage through physician-owned companies, but these policies usually carry practice restrictions and are far more expensive than group-sponsored insurance. In New York and Texas, ACNM successfully lobbied state legislators to extend joint underwriting authority to nurse-midwives. However, the premiums for this type of insurance are prohibitively expensive (in New York, the annual premium was $72,000, whereas the average CNM's annual salary is $25,000).

In July 1985, the ANA attempted to include nurse-midwives under its personal/professional liability insurance policy for all registered nurses. Under the current plan, nurses are protected for up to $1 million per claim and $3 million each year in total claims, and the policy covers all nurses practicing within the scope of their state's nurse practice act, including nurses in expanded practice roles. The cost of this coverage is low, because the risk is spread over a large group of nurses. The ANA believed that incorporation of the nurse-midwives into a larger policy was the optimal way to resolve the crisis, because of the importance of nurse-midwifery to nursing.

The coverage was marketed to the CNM population to enthusiastic acceptance. On August 30, however, ANA was informed by their insurance broker that the insurance company would exclude nurse-midwives from the policy. ANA was able to negotiate an agreement whereby CNMs could sign up for coverage until November 1, 1985, and all existing contracts would be honored for their one-year duration.

On September 19, 1985, ACNM and ANA testified about the insurance crisis before the Subcommittee on Commerce, Transportation, and Tourism of the House Committee on Energy and Commerce. They requested that Congress authorize a federally sponsored temporary program to provide reinsurance to a private insurance company providing liability insurance for nurse-midwives. The testimony before the committee by both organizations emphasized the low rate of claims, cost-effectiveness, and benefits to medically underserved communities associated with nurse-midwifery practice.

As of November 1985, ACNM felt that it had several choices still open. Its first choice was to set up its own insurance company: in other words, for nurse-midwives to provide self-insurance for members of their profession, just as physicians do (half of malpractice policies are written by physician-owned companies). Second, the nurse-midwives might also pursue the option of attempting to secure reinsurance through the federal government for their insurance company. Third, the nurse-midwives could continue to work with the states to obtain joint underwriting authority. This process would be time-consuming because it would be necessary to go to each state individually; in addition, premiums might be high. Fourth, an attempt has been made to work through the Federal Trade Commission (FTC). The FTC works on restraint-of-trade issues. In this case they would be evaluating whether denial of insurance coverage constitutes restraint of trade.

In October 1985, the ACNM board of directors decided to give priority to the self-insurance option. Under this plan, an ACNM insurance program would be established. Thus the problem has come full circle, and the policy issue moves, at least in part, from the public domain back into the private sector.

At the same time, however, Congress is addressing the crisis in several ways. For example, the Senate Appropriations Committee included $1 million in its fiscal year 1986 appropriations bill for the Department of Health and Human Services to investigate the issue of professional liability insurance coverage, especially for nurse-midwives. Senator Daniel Inouye (D–Hawaii) recommended language for the bill that might allow the department to begin functioning immediately as a reinsurer for nurse-midwives. Other initiatives on the insurance problem have been taken or are to be taken in the Senate Commerce Committee, the House Subcommittee on Commerce, Transportation, and Tourism (the Sept. 19 hearings referred to above), and a presidential Insurance Task Force.

The issue is far from resolved, and it is an important one for all nurses to remain aware of and to keep their state and federal legislators informed about. There is a crisis, and the government has a role in it, even if it is only to study the matter. The current situation severely restricts the employment practice of a great many people. Even if a satisfactory solution for the nurse-midwives is reached, the situation will require ongoing monitoring and cooperation from public and private sectors to prevent a similar crisis from happening again.

Case Study Questions

1. To what do you attribute the nurse-midwives' success in gaining a place in the health care system? Consider both clinical, social, and organizational factors.
2. Explain the causes of and reactions to the nurse-midwives' insurance problems. List recent events that have changed the

situation as described in the case. Could the problems have been foreseen and forestalled?

3. Where does the responsibility for nurse-midwifery liability insurance lie? Within the government? In what branch, level, or agency? Do you agree that the government should have a role in ameliorating the crisis? Does responsibility lie in the private sector? With a professional organization or employer? Why?

4. What does this case teach other nurses with expanded practice roles? What preventive actions can they take?

5. What interest groups, both in health care and outside the health care field, would be instrumental as members of a coalition to make the nurse-midwives' request to Congress for reinsurance more effective?

6. Review the strategies the nurse-midwives have used so far. Which arguments have been effective, and with whom (government, consumers, the insurance industry)? Explain why they chose self-insurance over the other alternatives. How might they have improved their strategy?

7. Given the choice of the self-insurance route, what does a nurse-midwife in independent practice need to know before buying into the insurance policy? What information will the ACNM need to give to the public? What would a potential investor need to know about the company?

REFERENCES AND SUPPLEMENTARY READINGS

The Case Study Method

Applegate, M. L., & Entrekin, N. M. (1984). *Teaching Ethics in Nursing*. New York: National League for Nursing.

Berquist, W. H., & Phillips, S. R. (1981). Interaction-Based Instructional Methods. In *A Handbook for Faculty Development*, Vol. 3. Council of Independent Colleges.

Hanson, P. G. (1981). *Learning Through Groups*. San Diego, CA: University Associates, Inc.

Kolb, D. A. (1984). *Experiential Learning*. Englewood Cliffs, NJ: Prentice-Hall.

Lambert, L. (1984). *How Adults Learn: An Interview Study of Leading Researchers, Policy Makers and Staff Developers*. Paper presented at the American Educational Research Association, New Orleans.

Lynn, L. E. (1980). *Designing Public Policy: A Casebook on the Role of Policy Analysis.* Santa Monica, CA: Goodyear Publishing Company.

Rakich, J., Longest, J., & Darr, K. (1983). *Cases in Health Managment.* Philadelphia: W. B. Saunders.

Ronstadt, R. (1977). *The Art of Case Analysis.* Needhan: Lord Publishing.

Baby Doe

For further information about this issue, refer to the following sources. Also, use current information available at the time you analyze the case.

ANA and AACN criticize Baby Doe regulations. (March 1985). *Capital Update, 3,* 2.

Baby Doe legislation signed by President. (October 1985). *Capital Update, 2,* 7.

Committee on the Legal and Ethical Aspects of Health Care for Children. (1983). Comments and recommendations on the "Infant Doe" proposed regulations. *Law, Medicine and Health Care, 11,* 203–209, 213.

Conferees agree on Baby Doe legislation. (September 1984). *Capital Update, 2,* 2.

Doudera, A. (1983). Section 504, handicapped newborns, and ethics committees: An alternative to the hotline. *Law, Medicine and Health Care, 11,* 200–202, 236.

Drane, J. F. (January–February 1984). The defective child: Ethical guidelines for painful dilemmas. *JOGN Nursing, 13,* 42–48.

Feldman, E., & Murray, T. H. (1984). State legislation and the handicapped newborn: A moral and political dilemma. *Law, Medicine and Health Care, 12,* 156–163.

Final Baby Doe regulations published. (April 1985). *Capital Update, 3,* 4.

Lyon, J. (1985). *Playing God in the Nursery.* New York: W. W. Norton.

New Baby Doe rule cools controversy. (1984). *AORN Journal, 39,* 814–815.

Paris, J. J., & Fletcher, A. B. (1983). Infant Doe regulations and the absolute requirement to use nourishment and fluids for the dying infant. *Law, Medicine and Health Care, 11,* 210–213.

Solomon, S. (1984). Baby Doe cases raise questions about government role. *Nursing & Health Care, 5,* 238–239.

Nurse-Midwives

American College of Nurse-Midwives. (September 19, 1985). *Testimony on the scarcity and high cost of insurance.* Washington: American College of Nurse-Midwives.

American Nurses' Association. (September 19, 1985). *Testimony on the unavailability of liability insurance for nurse-midwives.* Washington: American Nurses' Association.

Bullough, B. (1985). Nurse midwifery. *Pediatric Nursing, 11,* 143–148.

Colburn, D. (July 3, 1985). Midwives face insurance crisis. *The Washington Post,* p. 7.

Krause, N. (1985). Supplemental report on nurse-midwifery legislation. *Journal of Nurse-Midwifery, 30,* 133–136.

Malpractice and midwives. (July 6, 1985). Editorial, *The Washington Post,* p. A18.

McCarthy, C. (July 21, 1985). Nurse-midwives and their struggle to survive. *The Washington Post,* p. B5.

Nurse-midwifery trends: Some reflections. (1985). *Journal of Nurse-Midwifery, 30,* 1–2.

Reforming malpractice law. (September 30, 1985). *Medicine & Health,* Perspectives.

Robinson, S. (1985). Role restrictions. *Nursing Times, 81,* 28–31.

Solomon, S. (1985). Diverse issues call for decisive action. *Nursing & Health Care, 6,* 479–480.

Solomon, S. (1985). D.C. regulatory battle proves our fight is far from over. *Nursing & Health Care, 6,* 242–243.